Ultimate Pocket Guide TO Lactation Management

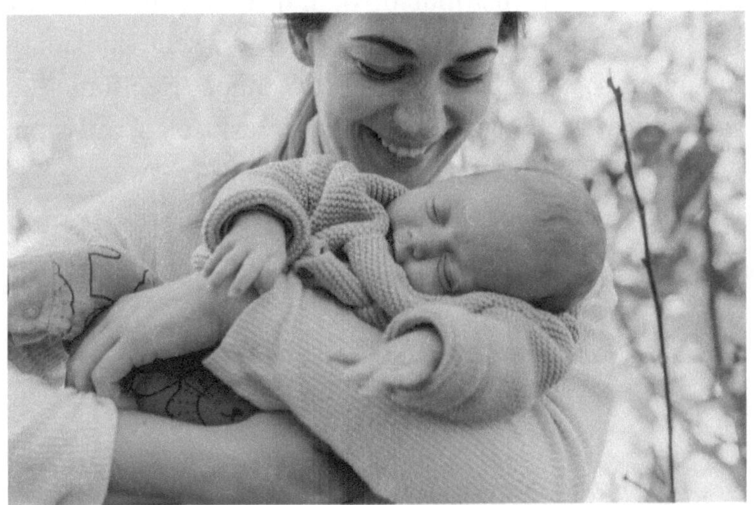

Enhance Breastfeeding Experience with Expert Advice

Dr. Veronica James

TABLE OF CONTENT

INTRODUCTION

Breastfeeding is a remarkable and natural process that not only nourishes infants but also creates an unbreakable bond between mothers and their babies. The act of breastfeeding provides a unique opportunity for mothers to connect with their little ones on a deeply intimate and emotional level. However, while breastfeeding is a beautiful and instinctual act, it can also present challenges and uncertainties for many mothers.

In this pocket guide, we delve into the world of lactation management, offering a comprehensive resource to support mothers on their breastfeeding journey. Whether you are an expectant mother preparing for the arrival of your little one or a new mother seeking guidance and reassurance, this guide aims to equip you with the knowledge, strategies, and tools necessary to overcome obstacles and achieve successful breastfeeding.

Within these pages, we explore the countless benefits of breastfeeding. From the optimal nutrition breast milk provides, tailored specifically to meet the needs of growing infants, to the powerful immunological advantages that protect babies against infections and diseases, breastfeeding is a gift that keeps on giving. Moreover, we shed light on the profound emotional connection that breastfeeding nurtures, fostering a sense of security, love, and attachment between mother and child.

Understanding the pivotal role that lactation consultants play in supporting breastfeeding journeys, we highlight the invaluable expertise they bring to the table. These dedicated healthcare professionals are equipped with the knowledge and skills to guide and empower mothers, addressing concerns, providing practical assistance, and offering emotional support. Whether it's assisting with latching techniques, resolving issues of low milk supply, or navigating breastfeeding challenges in unique circumstances, lactation consultants are there to help mothers thrive in their breastfeeding experience.

In this guide, we tackle common challenges and concerns faced by breastfeeding mothers. From addressing issues such as engorgement, nipple pain, and mastitis, to exploring strategies for managing an oversupply or coping with the demands of returning to work or school, we provide practical advice and evidence-based solutions. We also delve into special circumstances, including premature babies, multiples, and the impact of medications, ensuring that mothers facing unique challenges can find the guidance they need.

We understand that breastfeeding is not just a journey for mothers alone; it is a journey that involves partners, families, and communities. Recognizing the importance of a supportive environment, we delve into ways to involve partners and families in the breastfeeding process, provide resources for breastfeeding education, and explore strategies for overcoming social and cultural challenges that may arise.

Lastly, we explore the topic of weaning and extended breastfeeding, offering insights into signs of readiness for weaning, introducing solid foods, and navigating the emotional aspects of this transition. We also shed light on the benefits and considerations of extended breastfeeding, empowering mothers to make informed choices that align with their unique circumstances and desires.

Throughout this pocket guide, we aim to empower and support mothers, helping them embrace the transformative journey of breastfeeding with confidence and joy. By equipping mothers with knowledge, providing practical strategies, and fostering a sense of community, we hope to celebrate the beautiful bond that breastfeeding nurtures and encourage every mother to embark on this remarkable adventure with love, determination, and resilience.

CHAPTER 1

BENEFITS OF BREASTFEEDING

Breastfeeding is a remarkable journey that goes beyond providing nourishment to your baby. It is a unique and invaluable experience that offers a multitude of benefits for both infants and mothers. In this section, we explore the numerous advantages of breastfeeding, highlighting the extraordinary ways it supports the growth, development, and overall well-being of your baby.

Optimal Nutrition:

Breast milk is a living, dynamic substance that is perfectly designed to meet the nutritional needs of infants. It contains an ideal balance of proteins, carbohydrates, fats, vitamins, and minerals, all essential for healthy growth and development. The composition of breast milk changes as your baby grows, adapting to their specific needs at each stage.

Immunological Advantages:

Breast milk is rich in antibodies, immune cells, and other bioactive compounds that provide crucial protection against infections and diseases. It helps strengthen your baby's immune system, reducing the risk of respiratory infections, gastrointestinal illnesses, ear infections, and certain chronic conditions later in life.

Digestive Health:

Breast milk is easily digestible, which helps prevent constipation and reduces the likelihood of digestive issues in infants. It contains enzymes that aid digestion, promoting the development of a healthy gut microbiome and potentially reducing the risk of allergies and food intolerances.

Cognitive and Developmental Benefits:

The components of breast milk, including long-chain fatty acids and specific proteins, support optimal brain development and cognitive function in infants. Breastfeeding has been associated with improved IQ scores, enhanced memory, and better overall neurodevelopmental outcomes.

Bonding and Emotional Connection:

The act of breastfeeding fosters a profound emotional bond between mother and baby. Skin-to-skin contact, eye contact, and the release of oxytocin during breastfeeding promote feelings of love, comfort, and security, strengthening the emotional connection between you and your little one.

Reduced Risk of Chronic Diseases:

Breastfeeding has long-term health benefits for both infants and mothers. Breastfed babies have a lower risk of obesity, type 2 diabetes, asthma, allergies, and certain childhood cancers. Mothers who breastfeed have a reduced risk of breast and ovarian cancers, as well as cardiovascular disease and osteoporosis.

Postpartum Recovery:

Breastfeeding stimulates the release of hormones that promote uterine contractions, aiding in the recovery of the uterus after childbirth. It also helps in reducing postpartum bleeding and may assist with weight loss by burning extra calories.

Convenience and Cost-Effectiveness:

Breastfeeding eliminates the need for preparing bottles, sterilizing equipment, and buying formula, making it a convenient and cost-effective feeding option. Breast milk is readily available and always at the perfect temperature for your baby.

Environmental Sustainability:

Breastfeeding is an environmentally friendly choice. It generates no waste, requires no packaging, and has a minimal carbon footprint compared to the production, packaging, and transportation of formula.

The benefits of breastfeeding extend far beyond nutrition alone, encompassing physical health, emotional well-being, and environmental sustainability. By choosing to breastfeed, you are providing your baby with a powerful foundation for a healthy start in life while nurturing a beautiful bond that will last a lifetime.

ROLE OF LACTATION CONSULTANTS

Breastfeeding is a natural process, but it can also be a learned skill that requires support, guidance, and sometimes troubleshooting. This is where lactation consultants play a pivotal role. Lactation consultants are healthcare professionals with specialized knowledge and training in breastfeeding management. Their expertise and compassionate support are invaluable in helping mothers navigate the intricacies of breastfeeding and overcome challenges that may arise along the way. Let's explore the role of lactation consultants in greater detail.

Education and Counseling:

Lactation consultants provide essential education and counseling to expectant and new mothers. They equip mothers with evidence-based information about breastfeeding techniques, proper positioning and latch, understanding infant feeding cues, and establishing an adequate milk supply. This education empowers mothers to make informed decisions and build confidence in their breastfeeding journey.

Assessing and Promoting Optimal Latch and Milk Transfer:

Lactation consultants have the skills to assess breastfeeding techniques and identify any issues that may hinder proper latch or hinder the baby's ability to effectively transfer milk. They evaluate the latch, positioning, oral anatomy, and suck-swallow patterns to ensure efficient milk transfer and prevent problems like sore nipples, low milk supply, or ineffective sucking.

Troubleshooting Challenges:

Breastfeeding can come with challenges, such as engorgement, mastitis (breast infection), nipple pain or damage, and difficulties with milk supply. Lactation consultants are adept at identifying the underlying causes of these challenges and providing appropriate interventions and strategies. They offer practical solutions tailored to each mother's unique circumstances, helping to resolve issues and improve the overall breastfeeding experience.

Specialized Care for Complex Situations:

Lactation consultants are particularly valuable when faced with specialized situations or complex breastfeeding challenges. For example, if a baby is born prematurely, has a medical condition, or requires neonatal intensive care, lactation consultants can offer specialized guidance on breastfeeding and pumping for these situations. They provide support and strategies to overcome obstacles and help mothers establish and maintain a breastfeeding relationship even in challenging circumstances.

Emotional Support:

Breastfeeding can be an emotional journey for mothers, filled with joy, but also moments of frustration, doubt, and fatigue. Lactation consultants recognize the emotional aspect of breastfeeding and provide a nurturing and non-judgmental space for mothers to express their concerns, fears, and questions. They offer empathy, reassurance, and emotional support, playing a crucial role in boosting mothers' confidence and helping them navigate the emotional challenges that may arise.

Collaborative Approach:

Lactation consultants work collaboratively with other healthcare providers, including obstetricians, pediatricians, nurses, and midwives. They communicate and share information to ensure comprehensive care and continuity throughout the mother's breastfeeding journey. This collaboration helps create a supportive network of professionals working together to optimize the breastfeeding experience for both mother and baby.

Ongoing Education and Advocacy:

Lactation consultants stay up-to-date with the latest research, guidelines, and best practices in lactation management. They continually update their knowledge and skills through professional development activities, enabling them to provide the most current and evidence-based care. Lactation consultants also serve as advocates for breastfeeding, promoting its importance within healthcare systems, communities, and public health initiatives.

The role of lactation consultants is multifaceted and encompasses education, assessment, troubleshooting, emotional support, and advocacy. Their expertise, combined with their passion for promoting successful breastfeeding, make them an invaluable resource for mothers and families. By working hand in hand with lactation consultants, mothers can overcome challenges, establish a positive breastfeeding experience, and nourish their babies with confidence and joy.

COMMON CHALLENGES AND CONCERNS

While breastfeeding is a natural process, it is not always without its challenges. Many mothers encounter common difficulties and concerns along their breastfeeding journey. Recognizing and addressing these challenges is essential for promoting successful breastfeeding and ensuring the well-being of both mother and baby. Let's explore some of the common challenges and concerns in breastfeeding and discuss strategies to overcome them.

Latching Difficulties:

Proper latch is crucial for effective milk transfer and preventing nipple pain or damage. Lactation consultants can assess latch techniques, provide guidance on positioning and support, and suggest adjustments to promote a deep latch. Techniques such as breast compression and nipple shields may be recommended in certain cases to assist with latching difficulties.

Sore or Damaged Nipples:

Sore or cracked nipples can make breastfeeding painful and challenging. Lactation consultants can help identify the underlying causes of nipple soreness, such as improper latch or positioning, and provide strategies for healing and pain relief. They may suggest techniques to improve latch, recommend nipple creams or ointments, and advise on proper breast care.

Engorgement:

Engorgement occurs when the breasts become overly full and firm, making it difficult for the baby to latch. Lactation consultants can guide mothers on techniques to relieve engorgement, such as warm compresses, gentle massage, and frequent breastfeeding or pumping. They can also provide strategies to manage milk supply and prevent recurrent engorgement.

Mastitis:

Mastitis is a breast infection that can cause flu-like symptoms, breast pain, and inflammation. Lactation consultants can help mothers identify the signs of mastitis and guide them on strategies to manage it effectively. This may include continuing to breastfeed, using warm compresses, practicing frequent nursing or pumping, and in some cases, antibiotics.

Low Milk Supply:

Some mothers may experience concerns about low milk supply. Lactation consultants can assess the situation, help identify potential causes of low supply, and provide strategies to increase milk production. They may recommend techniques such as frequent breastfeeding, breast compression, skin-to-skin contact, and pumping to stimulate milk supply.

Oversupply and Fast Let-Down:

Conversely, some mothers may face issues with oversupply of milk, leading to a fast let-down reflex. This can cause discomfort for the baby, difficulty latching, or excessive spit-up. Lactation consultants can provide guidance on managing oversupply, including techniques to regulate milk flow, such as block feeding or expressing milk before feeding.

Breastfeeding and Work or School Commitments:

Balancing breastfeeding with work or school commitments can be a concern for many mothers. Lactation consultants can help mothers plan for successful breastfeeding while returning to work or school. They can provide guidance on pumping, milk storage, maintaining milk supply, and navigating workplace accommodations or breastfeeding-friendly environments.

Breastfeeding Twins or Multiples:

Mothers of twins or multiples may face unique challenges in breastfeeding. Lactation consultants can offer guidance on positioning, managing simultaneous breastfeeding, optimizing milk supply, and strategies to ensure adequate nutrition for all babies.

Breastfeeding and Medications:

Many mothers have concerns about the safety of breastfeeding while taking medications. Lactation consultants can provide information about medication compatibility with breastfeeding, assess potential risks, and offer guidance on medication choices that are safe for both mother and baby.

Emotional and Psychological Concerns:

Breastfeeding can bring about a range of emotions and psychological concerns for mothers, including feelings of guilt, anxiety, or postpartum depression. Lactation consultants play a crucial role in providing emotional support, reassurance, and referrals to appropriate resources when needed.

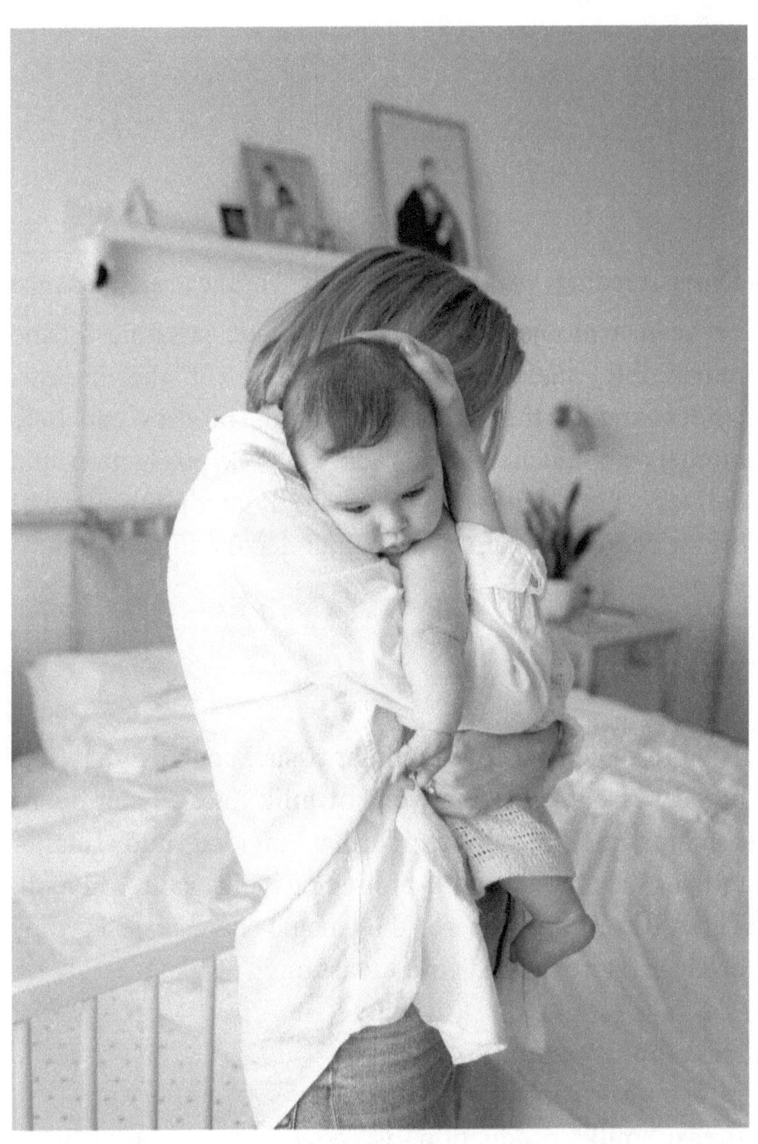

CHAPTER 2

ANATOMY AND PHYSIOLOGY OF BREASTFEEDING

Breastfeeding is a beautifully orchestrated dance between a mother and her baby, made possible by the remarkable anatomy and physiology of the breasts. Understanding the intricacies of this process can help mothers appreciate the miracle of milk production and delivery. Let's delve into the anatomy and physiology of breastfeeding to gain a deeper understanding of how it all works.

Breast Structure:

The breast consists of glandular tissue, connective tissue, blood vessels, and a network of milk ducts. Each breast contains multiple lobes, further divided into smaller lobules that house milk-producing cells called alveoli. The alveoli are where the magic happens, as they produce, store, and release breast milk.

Hormonal Regulation:

Breast milk production is governed by a delicate interplay of hormones. During pregnancy, the levels of estrogen and progesterone rise, preparing the breasts for milk production. After childbirth, the hormone prolactin stimulates the alveoli to produce milk, while oxytocin triggers the let-down reflex, causing the milk to flow.

Milk Production:

The production of breast milk is a supply-and-demand process. When a baby feeds at the breast, the stimulation from suckling triggers a release of prolactin, signaling the alveoli to produce milk. The more frequently and effectively the baby feeds, the more milk the breasts will produce to meet the demand. This is why establishing a good latch and nursing on demand are essential for maintaining an ample milk supply.

Let-Down Reflex:

The let-down reflex, also known as milk ejection reflex, is a crucial step in breastfeeding. It is triggered by the release of oxytocin, which causes the muscles around the alveoli to contract, squeezing the milk out of the breast and into the milk ducts. This reflex can be stimulated by the baby's suckling, the sound or sight of the baby, or even by feelings of love and relaxation.

Milk Composition:

Breast milk is a complex and dynamic fluid, tailored perfectly to meet the nutritional needs of a growing baby. It contains an ideal balance of proteins, carbohydrates, fats, vitamins, minerals, enzymes, and antibodies. The composition of breast milk changes throughout the feeding, with the initial milk, called foremilk, being more watery and thirst-quenching, followed by hindmilk, which is richer in fats and provides satiety.

Supply and Demand:

Breast milk production operates on a supply-and-demand principle. The more frequently and effectively a baby nurses, the more milk the breasts will produce to match the demand. On the other hand, if milk is not effectively removed from the breasts, whether due to infrequent feedings or improper latch, it can signal the body to decrease milk production. Establishing a good breastfeeding routine and nursing on demand are essential for maintaining an adequate milk supply.

Breast Engorgement and Milk Removal:

Engorgement, a common concern for breastfeeding mothers, occurs when the breasts become overly full and firm due to an abundance of milk. Regular breastfeeding or pumping sessions help remove milk from the breasts, preventing engorgement and promoting milk flow. Techniques such as breast compression and warm compresses can aid in milk removal and alleviate discomfort.

Breastfeeding Positions:

There are various breastfeeding positions that allow for comfortable and effective milk transfer. Some common positions include the cradle hold, cross-cradle hold, football hold, and side-lying position. Each position offers different benefits and may be suitable for different situations or preferences. Lactation consultants can provide guidance on finding the most comfortable and effective position for both mother and baby.

Understanding the intricate anatomy and physiology of breastfeeding enhances our appreciation for the incredible process of milk production and delivery. By

BREAST STRUCTURE AND MILK PRODUCTION

The breasts are a remarkable part of a woman's anatomy, designed specifically to support the production and delivery of breast milk. Understanding the structure and function of the breasts is fundamental to comprehending the process of milk production. Let's explore the key aspects of breast structure and how milk is produced.

Breast Anatomy:

The breasts are composed of glandular tissue, connective tissue, blood vessels, and a network of milk ducts. Each breast contains multiple lobes, and within each lobe, there are smaller structures called lobules. The lobules are composed of milk-producing cells called alveoli. These alveoli are the primary sites of milk synthesis and storage.

Milk Production:

Milk production, also known as lactogenesis, is a complex process regulated by hormones. During pregnancy, the breasts undergo significant changes in preparation for lactation. The hormones estrogen and progesterone, primarily produced by the ovaries and later by the placenta, stimulate the growth and development of the milk-producing structures in the breasts.

After childbirth, a shift in hormone levels occurs. The decrease in progesterone and the release of prolactin, a hormone secreted by the pituitary gland, trigger the initiation of milk production. Prolactin stimulates the alveoli to produce milk. The more frequently and effectively the breasts are emptied through breastfeeding or pumping, the more milk the breasts will produce to meet the demand.

Let-Down Reflex:

The let-down reflex, also known as the milk ejection reflex, is a crucial step in breastfeeding. It is the process by which milk is released from the alveoli and flows through the milk ducts to the nipple, making it available for the baby to consume. The let-down reflex is triggered by the hormone oxytocin.

Stimulated by the baby's suckling or other sensory cues associated with breastfeeding, oxytocin is released from the pituitary gland into the bloodstream. This hormone causes the muscles surrounding the alveoli to contract, squeezing the milk into the milk ducts and ultimately to the nipple. The let-down reflex can also be influenced by emotions, such as feelings of love and relaxation.

Milk Composition:

Breast milk is a dynamic and complex fluid, specifically tailored to meet the nutritional and developmental needs of a baby. Its composition changes throughout a feeding and as the baby grows. Breast milk contains a combination of proteins, carbohydrates, fats, vitamins, minerals, enzymes, hormones, and antibodies.

The initial milk that a baby receives during a feeding is called foremilk. Foremilk is relatively low in fat but provides hydration and quenches the baby's thirst. As the feeding progresses, the milk transitions to hindmilk, which is richer in fats and provides essential calories for the baby's growth and satiety.

Supply and Demand:

Breast milk production operates on a supply-and-demand principle. The more frequently and effectively the breasts are stimulated through breastfeeding or pumping, the more milk the breasts will produce to match the demand. On the other hand, if milk is not regularly and adequately removed from the breasts, it can signal the body to decrease milk production.

Establishing a good breastfeeding routine, feeding on demand, and ensuring proper latch and effective milk removal are key factors in maintaining an adequate milk supply.

In conclusion, the structure of the breasts, including the glandular tissue and milk ducts, along with the hormonal regulation of milk production, lay the foundation for successful lactation. Understanding the intricate processes of milk synthesis, the let-down reflex, and the dynamic composition of breast milk empowers mothers to navigate breastfeeding with confidence and provide optimal nutrition for their babies.

colostrum. Colostrum is rich in antibodies, proteins, vitamins, and minerals, providing essential immune protection and nutrition for the newborn.

HORMONAL INFLUENCES ON LACTATION

The process of lactation, or milk production, is regulated by a complex interplay of hormones that ensure the successful nourishment of an infant. These hormones orchestrate various physiological changes within the breast to support the production, release, and maintenance of breast milk. Let's explore the key hormones involved in lactation and their influences on this remarkable process.

Prolactin:

Prolactin is the primary hormone responsible for stimulating milk production in the breasts. It is produced and released by the anterior pituitary gland in response to the suckling or nipple stimulation during breastfeeding. Prolactin acts on the milk-producing cells within the alveoli of the mammary glands, promoting their growth, differentiation, and milk synthesis. The level of prolactin in the bloodstream increases during pregnancy and remains elevated after childbirth to support ongoing milk production. Frequent and effective breastfeeding or pumping sessions help maintain high prolactin levels, ensuring an ample milk supply for the baby.

Oxytocin:

Oxytocin is often referred to as the "love hormone" due to its role in social bonding and maternal-infant attachment. In the context of lactation, oxytocin plays a crucial role in the milk ejection reflex, also known as the let-down reflex. When a baby suckles at the breast or nipple stimulation occurs, oxytocin is released from the posterior pituitary gland. This hormone acts on the myoepithelial cells surrounding the alveoli, causing them to contract and squeeze the milk out of the alveoli into the milk ducts. The milk then flows through the ducts and is made available for the baby to consume. Oxytocin release is facilitated by feelings of love, relaxation, and positive emotions, creating a nurturing and bonding experience between the mother and her baby.

Estrogen and Progesterone:

Estrogen and progesterone, known as the pregnancy hormones, play essential roles in preparing the breasts for lactation during pregnancy. Estrogen promotes the growth and development of the milk ducts and stimulates the proliferation of mammary gland cells. Progesterone helps maintain the structure of the alveoli and stimulates the development of lobules within the breasts. Together, these hormones support the structural changes necessary for milk production.

Following childbirth, there is a rapid decline in estrogen and progesterone levels, which triggers the release of prolactin and initiates milk production. During lactation, the levels of estrogen and progesterone remain relatively low to facilitate sustained milk production. These hormones also have inhibitory effects on the milk ejection reflex, allowing the mother to breastfeed without milk flow occurring continuously.

Thyroid Hormones:

Thyroid hormones, including thyroxine (T4) and triiodothyronine (T3), are involved in regulating metabolism and energy balance in the body. They also play a role in lactation. Low levels of thyroid hormones can affect milk production and let-down reflex. Mothers with thyroid disorders may experience challenges in establishing and maintaining milk supply. It is important for women with thyroid conditions to work closely with their healthcare provider to ensure optimal thyroid hormone levels for successful lactation.

Cortisol and Stress Hormones:

Stress can have an impact on lactation and milk production. High levels of stress hormones, such as cortisol, can interfere with the release of oxytocin and disrupt the let-down reflex. Stress can also affect milk supply, milk composition, and breastfeeding behaviors. Therefore, creating a calm and supportive breastfeeding environment, managing stress levels, and seeking support are important for successful breastfeeding.

Understanding the hormonal influences on lactation helps mothers and healthcare professionals appreciate the

MILK EJECTION REFLEX

The Milk Ejection Reflex (MER), also known as the let-down reflex, is a physiological process that enables the release of breast milk from the alveoli into the milk ducts, making it available for the baby to consume during breastfeeding. The MER is essential for successful breastfeeding and plays a vital role in ensuring that the baby receives an adequate milk supply. Let's explore the milk ejection reflex in more detail.

Triggering the Milk Ejection Reflex:

The milk ejection reflex is initiated by the hormone oxytocin. Oxytocin is produced in the hypothalamus, a region of the brain, and stored in the posterior pituitary gland. It is released in response to specific stimuli, primarily the baby's suckling or nipple stimulation. Oxytocin release can also be triggered by other sensory cues associated with breastfeeding, such as the sight, sound, or smell of the baby, or even feelings of love and relaxation.

The Process of Milk Ejection:

When the baby latches onto the breast and begins to suckle, nerve signals are sent from the nipple to the hypothalamus. These signals stimulate the release of oxytocin from the posterior pituitary gland into the bloodstream. Oxytocin then travels through the bloodstream and reaches the mammary glands, where it acts on the myoepithelial cells surrounding the alveoli.

The myoepithelial cells respond to oxytocin by contracting rhythmically. This contraction exerts pressure on the alveoli, squeezing the milk within them and causing it to be pushed into the milk ducts. The milk flows through the ducts towards the nipple, where it can be readily available for the baby to feed.

The Sensation of Milk Ejection:

Many breastfeeding mothers experience a distinct sensation during the milk ejection reflex. This sensation can vary from person to person and may be described as tingling, warmth, or a gentle pulling or tugging sensation deep within the breast. Some mothers may not feel any specific sensation, which is also normal. The sensation is generally temporary and subsides once the milk is flowing smoothly.

Factors Affecting the Milk Ejection Reflex:

Several factors can influence the milk ejection reflex, either enhancing or inhibiting its response:

- **Emotional State**: Positive emotions, relaxation, and feelings of love can enhance the release of oxytocin and facilitate the milk ejection reflex. Conversely, stress, anxiety, and tension can hinder the reflex.
- **Distractions:** A calm and quiet environment during breastfeeding can help mothers focus on the breastfeeding experience and facilitate the milk ejection reflex. Excessive noise, distractions, or interruptions can disrupt the reflex.
- **Hormonal Imbalances:** Hormonal imbalances, such as low oxytocin levels or elevated stress

hormones, can impact the milk ejection reflex. It is important to address any underlying hormonal issues with the guidance of a healthcare professional.

- **Previous Breast Surgery or Trauma**: Certain breast surgeries or past trauma may affect the nerves and milk ducts, potentially impacting the milk ejection reflex. Lactation consultants can provide support and guidance for mothers who have had previous breast surgery or trauma.

Promoting a Healthy Milk Ejection Reflex:

To promote a healthy milk ejection reflex, it is important for mothers to create a comfortable and relaxing breastfeeding environment. Finding a quiet and peaceful space, minimizing distractions, and adopting relaxation techniques can help enhance the release of oxytocin and facilitate the milk ejection reflex. Establishing a positive breastfeeding relationship with the baby, ensuring a proper latch, and responding to the baby's feeding cues also contribute to a smooth milk ejection reflex.

Lactation consultants and breastfeeding support professionals can provide valuable guidance and support to mothers experiencing difficulties with the milk ejection reflex. They can offer techniques

CHAPTER 3

ESTABLISHING SUCCESSFUL BREASTFEEDING

Establishing successful breastfeeding is a crucial goal for new mothers, as it provides numerous benefits for both the baby and the mother. Breast milk is a complete and personalized source of nutrition, offering optimal growth, development, and immune protection for the baby. Moreover, breastfeeding promotes bonding, enhances maternal-infant attachment, and contributes to the overall health and well-being of both mother and child. Let's explore some key factors that contribute to establishing successful breastfeeding.

Early Initiation:

Initiating breastfeeding as early as possible after birth sets the stage for successful breastfeeding. Early skin-to-skin contact between the mother and the baby stimulates the release of hormones, such as oxytocin, that promote bonding and trigger the milk ejection reflex. It also allows the baby to root and find the breast, leading to the first breastfeeding session.

Proper Latch:

A proper latch is essential for effective breastfeeding. It ensures that the baby is able to effectively extract milk from the breast and stimulates milk production. To achieve a good latch, the baby's mouth should be wide open, with the lips flanged outward, encompassing a significant portion of the areola. The baby's chin should be pressed against the breast, and the tongue should be extended over the lower gum. Seeking guidance from a lactation consultant or breastfeeding specialist can be helpful in achieving and maintaining a proper latch.

Feeding on Demand:

Breastfed babies thrive on demand feeding, meaning they are fed whenever they show hunger cues, such as rooting, licking their lips, or sucking on their hands. Feeding on demand helps establish a good milk supply, ensures the baby receives sufficient nourishment, and promotes a healthy breastfeeding relationship. Newborns typically feed frequently, often every 2 to 3 hours, including during the night. As the baby grows, the feeding pattern may become more predictable and spaced out.

Positioning and Comfort:

Finding comfortable and supportive breastfeeding positions is important for both the mother and the baby.

There are various positions to try, such as the cradle hold, football hold, or side-lying position, depending on the mother's comfort and the baby's preference. Using pillows or nursing cushions can provide additional support. It's important to ensure that the baby's body is facing the mother, with the baby's ear, shoulder, and hip aligned. Comfortable positioning contributes to a relaxed and enjoyable breastfeeding experience.

Proper Nutrition and Hydration:

A well-nourished and hydrated mother is better equipped to produce an adequate milk supply. It is essential for breastfeeding mothers to prioritize their own nutrition and hydration. Eating a balanced diet, rich in fruits, vegetables, whole grains, lean proteins, and healthy fats, provides the necessary nutrients for milk production. Drinking plenty of water throughout the day is also important to maintain hydration.

Seek Support:

Breastfeeding can come with its challenges, and seeking support is crucial for success. Lactation consultants, breastfeeding support groups, and healthcare professionals can offer guidance, answer questions, and provide reassurance. They can address concerns such as low milk supply, nipple soreness, or difficulties with latch, and offer practical tips and strategies for overcoming obstacles.

Patience and Persistence:

Establishing successful breastfeeding takes time and patience. It is important to remember that both the mother and the baby are learning and adjusting to the breastfeeding process. It's normal to experience some challenges along the way, but with patience, persistence, and support, most obstacles can be overcome. Building a breastfeeding relationship requires time and practice.

Breastfeeding is a journey that evolves as the baby grows. It is important for mothers to trust their instincts, listen to their baby's cues, and embrace the unique breastfeeding

POSITIONING AND LATCH TECHNIQUES

Positioning and latch techniques are crucial for successful breastfeeding, as they ensure the baby can effectively extract milk from the breast and promote optimal milk transfer. A proper latch and comfortable positioning also help prevent nipple soreness and encourage a positive breastfeeding experience for both the mother and the baby. Let's explore some commonly used positioning and latch techniques:

Cradle Hold:

The cradle hold is one of the most common breastfeeding positions. To do this:
- Sit in a comfortable chair with good back support.
- Hold the baby in the crook of your arm on the side that you will be breastfeeding.
- Support the baby's head and neck with your hand, with their nose level with the nipple.
- Bring the baby's body close to yours, with their tummy against your tummy.
- Align the baby's ear, shoulder, and hip in a straight line.
- Ensure the baby's mouth is wide open and covering a large portion of the areola.

Football Hold:

The football hold is useful for mothers who have had a cesarean birth, twins, or if the baby has difficulty latching in other positions. To do this:

- Sit in a chair with armrests or use a nursing pillow to support the baby.

- Position the baby on the same side you will be breastfeeding, with their legs tucked under your arm and their body facing towards you.
- Support the baby's head and neck with your hand, with their nose level with the nipple.
- Bring the baby close to your breast, ensuring their mouth is wide open and covering a large portion of the areola.

Side-Lying Position:

The side-lying position is useful for breastfeeding during nighttime or when both the mother and the baby want to lie down. To do this:

- Lie on your side, using pillows for support if needed.
- Position the baby next to you, facing your breast.
- Align the baby's nose level with the nipple.
- Support the baby's head and neck with your hand, guiding them to latch onto the breast.

Cross-Cradle Hold:

The cross-cradle hold is helpful for mothers who need more control during the latch or have a premature or small baby. To do this:

- Sit in a comfortable chair with good back support.
- Use the arm opposite to the breast you will be nursing on.
- Hold the baby's head with your hand, supporting their neck and shoulders.
- Bring the baby's body close to your breast, with their nose level with the nipple.
- Ensure the baby's mouth is wide open and covering a large portion of the areola.

Tips for Achieving a Good Latch:

- Wait for the baby to open their mouth wide before bringing them to the breast.
- Position the baby's lower lip and tongue to be below the nipple.
- Aim the nipple towards the roof of the baby's mouth.
- Allow the baby's chin to touch the breast, ensuring they have a deep latch.
- Look and listen for signs of effective sucking and swallowing, such as rhythmic jaw movement and audible swallowing.

If you are experiencing difficulties with positioning or latch, consider seeking support from a lactation consultant or breastfeeding specialist. They can provide personalized guidance, assess the latch, and offer techniques to improve breastfeeding comfort and effectiveness.

Remember, practice and patience are key in finding the positioning and latch technique that works best for you and your baby.

ASSESSING MILK TRANSFER

Assessing milk transfer during breastfeeding is important to ensure that the baby is receiving an adequate amount of milk and that breastfeeding is effective. While it may not be possible to measure the exact volume of milk transferred, there are several signs and indicators that can help assess milk transfer. Here are some ways to assess milk transfer during breastfeeding:

Baby's Weight Gain:

Monitoring the baby's weight gain over time is one of the most reliable indicators of successful milk transfer. Adequate weight gain suggests that the baby is receiving enough milk. It is normal for newborns to lose some weight in the first few days after birth, but they should start gaining weight steadily by the second week. Consult with a healthcare professional to ensure that the baby's weight gain is appropriate.

Swallowing Sounds and Patterns:

Listen for audible swallowing sounds while the baby is breastfeeding. Swallowing indicates that the baby is effectively extracting milk from the breast. Initially, the baby may have short, quick sucks followed by swallowing. As the milk flow increases, the baby's sucking pattern may become deeper and more rhythmic, with longer pauses for swallowing.

Satiety and Contentment:

Observe the baby's behavior after a breastfeeding session. A content and satisfied baby is a good indication that milk transfer was successful. Signs of satiety include the baby appearing relaxed, content, and releasing the breast on their own when finished. If the baby is calm, content, and has a relaxed body posture after feeding, it suggests that they have received enough milk.

Diaper Output:

Monitoring the baby's diaper output can provide insights into milk transfer. In the first few days, the baby will have meconium stools, which are thick, dark, and sticky. As milk intake increases, the baby should have frequent wet diapers (at least 6-8 per day) and transition to yellow, seedy, breast milk stools by the fourth or fifth day. Adequate wet and dirty diapers suggest that the baby is getting enough milk.

Breast Fullness and Softening:

Pay attention to changes in breast fullness before and after breastfeeding. Initially, the breasts may feel full and firm before a feeding and softer after breastfeeding. This change in breast fullness indicates that milk is being transferred and consumed by the baby.

Breast Compression:

Using breast compression techniques during breastfeeding can help assess milk transfer. After the initial let-down, gently compress the breast with your hand while the baby is still latched. If you observe additional milk flow and swallowing, it indicates that there is more milk available and being transferred to the baby.

Seeking Professional Support:

If you have concerns about milk transfer or suspect that the baby is not getting enough milk, seek support from a lactation consultant or healthcare professional. They can evaluate breastfeeding technique, assess the baby's latch, and provide guidance and support to ensure optimal milk transfer.

Remember, breastfeeding is a dynamic process, and milk transfer can vary throughout the breastfeeding journey. If you have any concerns or questions, reach out to a healthcare professional or lactation consultant for personalized guidance and support.

NEWBORN FEEDING CUES

Newborns communicate their hunger and readiness to feed through various feeding cues. Recognizing these cues is important for responsive feeding and ensuring that the baby receives timely and adequate nutrition. Here are some common newborn feeding cues to watch for:

Rooting Reflex:

When a newborn's cheek is gently stroked or touched, they will instinctively turn their head toward the stimulus and open their mouth in search of the breast or a bottle nipple. This reflex is called the rooting reflex and is a clear sign that the baby is ready to feed.

Sucking Movements:

Babies may exhibit sucking movements with their lips, tongue, or fingers when they are hungry. They may suck on their fists, fingers, or even their own tongue. These repetitive sucking motions indicate their desire for nourishment.

Increased Alertness and Activity:

When babies are hungry, they tend to become more alert and active. They may wake up from sleep or become more fidgety, moving their arms and legs more vigorously. This increased alertness and restlessness can be a sign that they are seeking a feeding.

Mouthing and Licking:

Newborns may show an increased interest in mouthing and licking objects, such as their own hands, blankets, or even their caregiver's shoulder. This behavior is often a precursor to feeding and indicates their readiness to suckle.

Smacking or Licking Lips:

Babies may smack their lips or lick their lips in anticipation of feeding. This action can be accompanied by making sucking noises or movements with their mouth.

Crying:

Crying is a late hunger cue and indicates that the baby is very hungry. It is important to recognize earlier feeding cues before the baby reaches this stage of hunger. Crying is a way for babies to communicate their needs, including hunger, and should be responded to promptly.

It is important to note that every baby is unique, and feeding cues may vary slightly from one baby to another. Additionally, newborns have small stomach capacities, so they may require frequent feedings, often every 2 to 3 hours, including during the night.

By observing and responding to these feeding cues, caregivers can ensure that the baby's hunger is met promptly, leading to a more relaxed and effective feeding experience. Responsive feeding, where the baby is fed on demand rather than on a strict schedule, helps establish a healthy breastfeeding relationship and supports the baby's nutritional needs.

SKIN-TO-SKIN CONTACT AND KANGAROO CARE

Skin-to-skin contact and kangaroo care are two powerful practices that promote the well-being of newborns and their parents. These techniques involve placing the baby directly against the parent's bare skin, providing numerous benefits for both the baby and the caregiver. Let's explore these practices in more detail:

Skin-to-Skin Contact:

Skin-to-skin contact, also known as "kangaroo care," involves placing the naked baby (excluding the diaper) directly on the parent's bare chest. Here are the benefits of skin-to-skin contact:

- **Promotes Bonding**: Skin-to-skin contact fosters a deep emotional bond between the baby and the caregiver. The close physical proximity helps establish a sense of security and trust, enhancing the emotional connection.
- **Regulates Body Temperature**: Newborns are not yet fully capable of regulating their body temperature. Skin-to-skin contact helps maintain the baby's body temperature within the optimal range by utilizing the parent's warmth. It is especially beneficial for premature or low-birth-weight babies.
- **Supports Breastfeeding**: Skin-to-skin contact immediately after birth or during breastfeeding stimulates the release of hormones, such as oxytocin, which promotes milk production and

the let-down reflex. It also helps the baby locate the breast and facilitates the establishment of a successful breastfeeding relationship.

- **Stabilizes Heart Rate and Respiratory Rate:** Skin-to-skin contact has been shown to stabilize the baby's heart rate and respiratory rate, promoting physiological stability.
- **Reduces Stress and Crying**: Being in close contact with the parent's skin has a calming effect on the baby, reducing stress and soothing distress. This can result in decreased crying and increased overall contentment.

Kangaroo Care:

Kangaroo care is an extension of skin-to-skin contact that involves prolonged periods of holding the baby against the parent's bare chest. The baby is typically positioned upright, with their head supported and their legs flexed. Here are the benefits of kangaroo care:

- **Enhanced Parent-Infant Bonding:** Kangaroo care allows for longer periods of uninterrupted skin-to-skin contact, fostering a deep and intimate bond between the parent and the baby.
- **Improved Sleep Patterns:** The comforting closeness of kangaroo care has been shown to promote better sleep patterns in newborns.

Babies who experience kangaroo care often have more settled sleep and spend less time in a fussy or agitated state.

- **Regulation of Body Functions**: Kangaroo care helps regulate the baby's physiological functions, including body temperature, heart rate, and breathing. The parent's body acts as a natural regulator, providing the optimal environment for the baby's well-being.
- **Positive Impact on Brain Development:** The sensory-rich experience of kangaroo care stimulates the baby's brain development and enhances cognitive and emotional development over time.

Both skin-to-skin contact and kangaroo care are recommended practices for all newborns, regardless of birth weight or health status. These practices can be initiated immediately after birth and continued for as long as desired or needed. They provide a nurturing and supportive environment for the baby's growth and development while strengthening the bond between the baby and their caregiver.

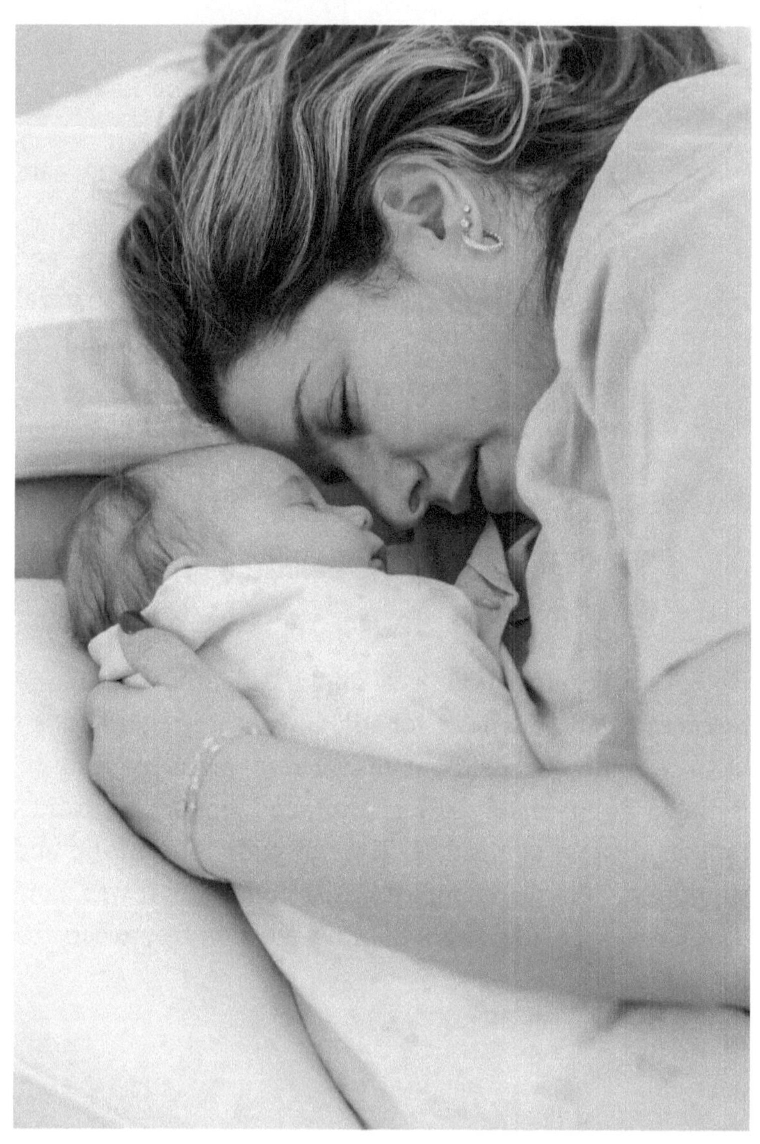

CHAPTER 4

EXPAND ON COMMON BREASTFEEDING DIFFICULTIES

Breastfeeding can bring immense joy and bonding between a mother and her baby, but it can also present challenges. Here are some common breastfeeding difficulties that mothers may encounter and strategies to address them:

Sore or Cracked Nipples:

Sore or cracked nipples are a common concern, especially in the early days of breastfeeding. They can occur due to an improper latch, positioning issues, or sensitivity to breastfeeding. To alleviate this problem:

- **Ensure a proper latch:** Position the baby correctly, aiming for a deep latch with the baby's mouth covering a large portion of the areola. Seek assistance from a lactation consultant if needed.
- **Break the latch gently:** Insert a clean finger into the corner of the baby's mouth to break the suction before removing the baby from the breast.

- **Apply nipple ointment:** Use a lanolin-based nipple ointment or breast milk to soothe and promote healing of cracked nipples.
- **Allow nipples to air dry:** After each feeding, expose the nipples to air to aid in healing. Avoid using harsh soaps or lotions on the nipples.

Engorgement:

Engorgement occurs when the breasts become excessively full and swollen due to an increase in milk production. This can make latching difficult for the baby. To manage engorgement:

- **Nurse frequently:** Breastfeed your baby on demand, ensuring that the breasts are emptied regularly to alleviate discomfort.
- **Apply warm compresses:** Prior to breastfeeding, apply warm compresses to the breasts to encourage milk flow and relieve engorgement.
- **Express milk:** If the baby is having difficulty latching due to severe engorgement, express a small amount of milk by hand or with a breast pump to soften the breast before offering it to the baby.
- **Cold packs:** Apply cold packs or chilled cabbage leaves to the breasts between feedings to reduce swelling and discomfort.

Low Milk Supply:

Some mothers may perceive their milk supply as low, leading to concerns about the baby not getting enough milk. It's important to remember that most mothers produce enough milk for their baby's needs. To address perceived low milk supply:

- **Nurse frequently and on demand:** Frequent breastfeeding stimulates milk production. Allow the baby to nurse whenever they show hunger cues.
- **Ensure proper latch:** A good latch helps the baby effectively remove milk from the breast, promoting milk supply.
- **Practice breast compression:** During breastfeeding, gently compress the breast to encourage milk flow and ensure the baby receives more milk.
- **Seek support:** Consult with a lactation consultant or healthcare provider who can assess breastfeeding techniques, evaluate the baby's growth, and provide guidance on increasing milk supply if necessary.

Mastitis:

Mastitis is an infection that can occur when bacteria enter the breast tissue, causing inflammation and pain. Signs of mastitis include breast tenderness, swelling, redness, and flu-like symptoms. To manage mastitis:

- **Continue breastfeeding**: It's safe to continue breastfeeding while having mastitis, as it helps to drain the breast and resolve the infection.
- **Apply warm compresses**: Use warm compresses or take warm showers to alleviate pain and promote milk flow.
- **Rest and hydration**: Get plenty of rest, stay well-hydrated, and maintain a nutritious diet to support your recovery.
- **Antibiotics**: If the infection does not improve within 24-48 hours or symptoms worsen, consult a healthcare professional for possible antibiotic treatment.

Overactive Let-Down or Oversupply:

Some mothers may experience an overactive let-down or an oversupply of milk, which can lead to the baby choking, gagging, or pulling away during breastfeeding. To manage an overactive let-down:

- **Latch techniques**: Use laid-back breastfeeding positions, such as reclining slightly, to allow gravity to slow the flow

Engorgement and mastitis are two common breastfeeding complications that can cause discomfort and affect breastfeeding. Here's an expanded explanation of each:

Engorgement:

Engorgement occurs when the breasts become overly full and swollen with milk. It typically happens in the early postpartum period when milk production is adjusting to the baby's needs. Some common causes of engorgement include a delay in initiating breastfeeding, infrequent or ineffective breastfeeding, or abrupt weaning. Here's how to manage engorgement:

- **Frequent breastfeeding:** Nurse your baby frequently, at least 8 to 12 times a day, to help empty the breasts and relieve engorgement.
- **Ensure proper latch:** Make sure your baby is latching properly and emptying the breasts effectively. Seek assistance from a lactation consultant if needed.

- **Express milk:** If your baby is having difficulty latching due to severe engorgement, express a small amount of milk by hand or with a breast pump to soften the breast before offering it to the baby.
- **Apply warm compresses:** Prior to breastfeeding, applying warm compresses or taking a warm shower can help increase blood flow to the breasts, relieve discomfort, and encourage milk flow.
- **Cold packs or cabbage leaves:** After breastfeeding, applying cold packs or chilled cabbage leaves to the breasts can reduce swelling and provide relief.
- **Avoid tight clothing or bras:** Wearing loose, comfortable clothing and a well-fitting bra can help minimize discomfort and allow for better milk flow.

Mastitis:

Mastitis is an infection of the breast tissue that can occur when bacteria enter through a cracked or sore nipple. It often presents with symptoms such as breast pain, redness, warmth, and flu-like symptoms such as fever and body aches. Mastitis requires prompt attention and treatment to prevent complications. Here's how to manage mastitis:

- **Continue breastfeeding:** It is safe to continue breastfeeding or expressing milk during mastitis. In fact, it is crucial to continue emptying the affected breast frequently to help resolve the infection and maintain milk supply.
- **Rest and hydration:** Get plenty of rest, as fatigue can worsen mastitis symptoms. Stay well-hydrated by drinking plenty of fluids.
- **Apply warm compresses:** Use warm compresses or take warm showers to alleviate pain, promote milk flow, and reduce inflammation.
- **Breastfeed on the affected side first**: Start breastfeeding on the affected breast to ensure thorough drainage of milk and relieve congestion.
- **Antibiotics**: If mastitis symptoms persist or worsen, consult a healthcare professional. They may prescribe antibiotics to treat the infection. It's important to complete the full course of antibiotics as prescribed.
- **Pain relief**: Over-the-counter pain relievers such as acetaminophen or ibuprofen can help alleviate pain and reduce inflammation. Consult with a healthcare professional for appropriate recommendations.

In both engorgement and mastitis cases, seeking support from a lactation consultant or healthcare professional can provide personalized guidance and help ensure a successful breastfeeding experience. They can assess the situation, offer specific strategies, and monitor your progress to prevent complications and support your breastfeeding journey.

NIPPLE PAIN AND DAMAGE

Nipple pain and damage are common concerns that breastfeeding mothers may experience. It can range from mild discomfort to severe pain and can affect breastfeeding success. Here's an expanded explanation on nipple pain and damage, along with strategies to address them:

Nipple Pain:

Nipple pain during breastfeeding is often associated with an improper latch or positioning. The most common causes include:

- **Improper latch:** A shallow latch, where the baby primarily sucks on the nipple rather than taking in a good portion of the areola, can cause nipple pain. It's important to ensure a deep latch, with the baby's mouth covering a large portion of the areola.

- **Sensitive nipples:** Some women naturally have more sensitive nipples, which can lead to discomfort during breastfeeding. Over time, as the nipples toughen and adapt, the pain usually subsides.
- **Engorgement:** Engorgement can make breastfeeding more challenging and cause nipple pain. Ensuring frequent and effective breastfeeding can help alleviate this issue.

Strategies to address nipple pain include:

- **Seek help:** Consult with a lactation consultant to assess the latch and positioning, and to provide guidance on proper breastfeeding techniques.
- **Correct latch:** Ensure a deep latch, with the baby's mouth wide open and taking in a good portion of the areola. Break the suction gently before removing the baby from the breast.
- **Nursing positions:** Experiment with different breastfeeding positions to find the most comfortable and effective one for both you and your baby.
- **Nipple care:** Apply a lanolin-based nipple cream or breast milk to soothe and protect the nipples.

Avoid using soap or harsh products on the nipples, as they can further irritate the skin.

- **Express milk:** If the pain becomes too intense, consider using a breast pump to express milk and give your nipples a break while still providing breast milk to your baby.

Nipple Damage:

Nipple damage refers to cracks, blisters, or bleeding that can occur due to prolonged or severe nipple pain. It's crucial to address nipple damage promptly to prevent infection and ensure successful breastfeeding. Here's how to manage nipple damage:

- **Continue breastfeeding**: Despite nipple damage, it is generally safe to continue breastfeeding. The baby's saliva has healing properties, and breastfeeding helps stimulate milk production and maintain milk supply.
- **Improve latch:** Work with a lactation consultant to improve the latch and ensure the baby is effectively transferring milk. A proper latch can help prevent further damage and promote healing.
- **Air dry and nipple ointments**: After each feeding, allow the nipples to air dry to promote

healing. Apply a lanolin-based nipple ointment or breast milk to provide moisture and protection.

- **Breast shells or nipple shields**: In some cases, using breast shells or nipple shields may help protect damaged nipples and provide relief while breastfeeding. However, these should be used under the guidance of a lactation consultant.
- **Evaluate feeding equipment:** If using a breast pump, check that the flange size is appropriate and that the pump settings are not causing further discomfort or damage.
- **Pain relief:** Over-the-counter pain relievers such as acetaminophen or ibuprofen can help alleviate pain during the healing process. Consult with a healthcare professional for appropriate recommendations.

Remember, with proper support and adjustments, nipple pain and damage can be overcome. Don't hesitate to seek assistance from a lactation consultant or healthcare professional who can provide individualized guidance and support for your breastfeeding journey.

LOW MILK SUPPLY

Low milk supply is a concern that some breastfeeding mothers may experience. It can lead to feelings of frustration and worry about not providing enough nourishment for the baby. While most mothers produce an adequate milk supply for their babies, here are some factors that can contribute to low milk supply and strategies to address them:

Insufficient Breast Stimulation:

- **Frequent and Effective Breastfeeding**: Breastfeed your baby frequently, aiming for at least 8 to 12 nursing sessions in 24 hours. Ensure that each breastfeeding session is effective by ensuring a proper latch and allowing the baby to nurse for as long as they need.
- **Breast Compression:** During breastfeeding, gently compress the breast to encourage milk flow and ensure the baby is receiving more milk. This can be done by applying gentle pressure on the breast with your hand.
- **Offer Both Breasts**: Allow the baby to nurse on both breasts during each feeding to stimulate milk production.

Inadequate Milk Removal:

- **Empty the Breasts**: Ensure that the breasts are fully emptied during breastfeeding or pumping sessions. Encourage the baby to nurse on one breast until it feels soft and then offer the second breast.

- **Pumping after Nursing**: If there is concern about low milk supply, consider pumping after nursing to further stimulate milk production and increase milk supply.

Maternal Factors:

- Proper Nutrition and Hydration: Maintain a well-balanced diet and stay well-hydrated. Adequate fluid intake can support milk production.
- Rest and Stress Management: Get enough rest and manage stress levels. Fatigue and stress can negatively impact milk supply. Rest when the baby sleeps and seek support from family and friends.
- Skin-to-Skin Contact: Practice skin-to-skin contact with your baby, as it helps release hormones that promote milk production.

Seek Support:

- **Lactation Consultant**: Consult with a lactation consultant who can assess breastfeeding techniques, evaluate the baby's growth, and provide guidance on increasing milk supply if necessary.

- **Support Groups**: Join local breastfeeding support groups or online communities where you can connect with other breastfeeding mothers and gain support and advice.

Galactagogues:

- Herbal Remedies: Some herbs such as fenugreek, blessed thistle, and fennel are believed to have lactation-boosting properties. Consult with a healthcare professional before using any herbal remedies.
- Prescription Medications: In some cases, prescription medications like domperidone or metoclopramide may be prescribed to increase milk supply. Discuss this option with a healthcare professional.

Remember, the perception of low milk supply is common, but it's essential to consult with a healthcare professional or lactation consultant to evaluate the situation and provide appropriate guidance. They can help determine if there is a true issue with milk supply or if adjustments can be made to improve breastfeeding outcomes.

Oversupply and fast let-down are two related issues that some breastfeeding mothers may experience. While low milk supply is a concern for some, others may find that they have an oversupply of milk, which can present its own challenges. Here's an expanded explanation of oversupply and fast let-down, along with strategies to manage them:

Oversupply of Milk:

Oversupply occurs when a mother produces more milk than her baby needs for adequate nourishment. This can lead to a range of issues, including engorgement, discomfort for the mother, and difficulties for the baby in effectively latching and managing the milk flow. Here are some strategies to manage oversupply:

- **Block Feeding**: Rather than switching breasts during feedings, allow the baby to fully drain one breast before offering the other breast. This helps to balance the milk supply and reduce oversupply.
- **Express Milk**: If the breasts are excessively full and uncomfortable, consider expressing a small amount of milk before nursing to reduce the

forceful flow and make it easier for the baby to latch.

- **Reclined Nursing Positions**: Try breastfeeding while in a reclined position, as this can help slow down the milk flow and allow the baby to manage the milk more easily.
- **Burp During Feeding**: Burping the baby during feedings can help alleviate discomfort caused by swallowing air due to a forceful let-down.

Fast Let-Down:

Fast let-down refers to the rapid flow of milk that can occur at the start of breastfeeding. It can overwhelm the baby, causing coughing, choking, or pulling away from the breast. Here are some strategies to manage fast let-down:

- **Breast Compression**: Before nursing, gently compress the breast to slow down the flow of milk. This can be done by applying gentle pressure on the breast near the areola with your hand.
- **Laid-Back Breastfeeding**: Try reclining slightly while breastfeeding, allowing gravity to help slow down the flow of milk.
- **Switch Nursing**: If the flow is too fast for the baby, switch back and forth between breasts

during feedings to help regulate the flow and provide breaks for the baby.

- **Nursing Positions**: Experiment with different breastfeeding positions to find the one that works best for your baby. Some positions, such as side-lying or the football hold, may help manage fast let-down.

- **Burp During Feeding**: Burping the baby during feedings can help relieve any discomfort caused by swallowing air due to a fast let-down.

It's important to note that oversupply and fast let-down can improve over time as breastfeeding patterns establish and the baby becomes more efficient at nursing. However, if these issues persist or cause significant difficulties, it may be helpful to consult with a lactation consultant who can provide personalized guidance and support.

Remember, every breastfeeding journey is unique, and finding strategies that work for you and your baby is essential. Patience, support, and seeking professional guidance can make a significant difference in managing oversupply and fast let-down while maintaining a positive breastfeeding experience.

Jaundice is a common condition in newborns characterized by yellowing of the skin and eyes. It occurs when there is an excess of bilirubin, a yellow pigment produced during the breakdown of red blood cells, in the baby's blood. While jaundice can occur in breastfed and formula-fed babies alike, there are specific considerations related to breastfeeding and jaundice. Here's an expanded explanation of jaundice and its relationship with breastfeeding:

Breastfeeding and Jaundice:

Breastfeeding itself does not cause jaundice. In fact, breastfeeding is beneficial for the baby's overall health and immune system. However, jaundice can sometimes be more common or prolonged in breastfed babies due to a few factors:

- **Colostrum and Milk Production**: In the early days after birth, a mother's breasts produce colostrum, a thick, yellowish fluid rich in nutrients and antibodies. Colostrum acts as a natural laxative, helping the baby pass meconium (the first stool) and eliminate bilirubin from the body. However, it is lower in volume compared to mature breast milk, which can lead to a slower transition of stools and bilirubin elimination.

- **Feeding Frequency**: In the first few days, establishing a frequent feeding pattern is crucial. Frequent breastfeeding stimulates bowel movements and helps the baby eliminate bilirubin.
- **Effective Milk Transfer**: Ensuring a proper latch and effective milk transfer during breastfeeding is important. If the baby is not removing milk efficiently, it may contribute to inadequate stooling and slower elimination of bilirubin.

Managing Jaundice in Breastfed Babies:

Most cases of breastfeeding-associated jaundice are mild and resolve on their own as breastfeeding patterns become well-established. Here are some strategies to manage jaundice in breastfed babies:

- **Frequent Breastfeeding:** Ensure that you breastfeed your baby at least 8 to 12 times a day, offering both breasts during each feeding session. Frequent breastfeeding helps stimulate milk production, promote effective milk transfer, and increase bowel movements to eliminate bilirubin.

- **Proper Latch and Milk Transfer:** Work with a lactation consultant to ensure a good latch and effective milk transfer during breastfeeding. This ensures that the baby receives an adequate amount of milk and helps prevent or resolve any feeding difficulties that may contribute to jaundice.
- **Watch for Signs of Adequate Feeding:** Monitor your baby's feeding patterns and diaper output. Look for signs of sufficient milk intake, such as active sucking and swallowing during feeds, weight gain, and an adequate number of wet and soiled diapers.
- **Consult with Healthcare Professionals:** If your baby's jaundice appears severe, persists beyond two weeks, or is causing concern, consult with your healthcare provider. They can evaluate the situation, assess bilirubin levels, and recommend appropriate interventions if necessary.

It's important to remember that each baby's situation is unique, and the management of jaundice may vary. Your healthcare provider will guide you based on your baby's specific needs and bilirubin levels.

Overall, breastfeeding is highly encouraged even if your baby has jaundice. The benefits of breastfeeding far outweigh the risks associated with jaundice, and most cases of breastfeeding-associated jaundice can be managed with proper breastfeeding techniques and support.

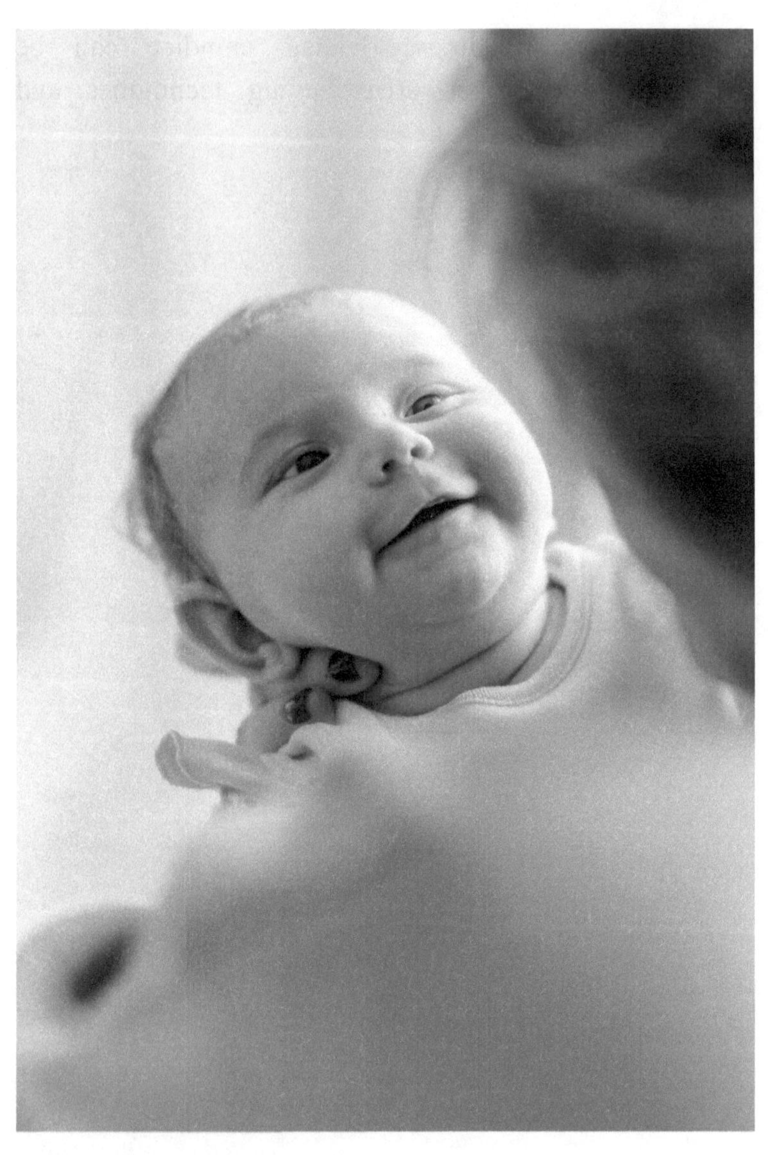

CHAPTER 5

MANAGING SPECIAL SITUATIONS

Managing special situations in lactation management requires specific considerations and adjustments to ensure successful breastfeeding. Here are expanded explanations for managing some common special situations:

Premature Babies:

Premature babies often face unique challenges when it comes to breastfeeding due to their immature sucking and swallowing reflexes. Here are strategies to support breastfeeding premature babies:

- **Kangaroo Care**: Practice kangaroo care, where the baby holds skin-to-skin against the mother's chest. This promotes bonding, regulates the baby's temperature, and enhances breastfeeding cues.
- **Pumping and Tube Feeding**: If the baby is unable to latch directly, express breast milk and provide it through a feeding tube to ensure they receive the benefits of breast milk.
- **Gradual Introduction to Breastfeeding**: Work closely with a lactation consultant to gradually

introduce breastfeeding as the baby grows and develops stronger sucking skills.

Twins or Multiples:

Breastfeeding twins or multiples can be demanding, but it is possible with the right support and strategies:

- **Tandem Feeding**: Feed both babies simultaneously by positioning them on each breast or using a combination of breast and bottle feeding to ensure they receive adequate nourishment.
- **Seek Help and Resources**: Connect with local breastfeeding support groups or seek guidance from a lactation consultant who has experience with multiples to learn effective positioning and feeding techniques.
- **Establish a Routine**: Create a feeding routine that works for you and your babies, ensuring they are fed at regular intervals and giving equal attention to each baby.

Maternal Medical Conditions or Medications:

Certain maternal medical conditions or medications may require special considerations for breastfeeding:

- **Consult with Healthcare Providers**: Consult with your healthcare provider or a lactation consultant to discuss any medical conditions or medications you may have. They can provide guidance on the safety of breastfeeding and recommend any necessary precautions or adjustments.
- **Medication Compatibility**: Ask your healthcare provider to assess the compatibility of medications with breastfeeding. In many cases, there are medications that can be safely used while breastfeeding, but dosage adjustments or alternative medications may be necessary.
- **Establishing Milk Supply**: If you're temporarily unable to breastfeed due to a medical condition or medication, regularly pump or hand express milk to establish and maintain milk supply until you can resume breastfeeding.

Adoption or Surrogacy:

Breastfeeding is still possible for parents who adopt or use surrogacy. Although lactation may not occur naturally, there are options to induce lactation or provide supplemental feeding:

- **Induced Lactation:** Work with a lactation consultant to develop a plan for induced lactation, which may involve hormone therapy, pumping, and using supplemental nursing systems to encourage milk production and bonding.

- **Supplemental Feeding**: In cases where full lactation is not possible, supplemental nursing systems or using donor milk can help provide the benefits of breastfeeding while ensuring the baby receives adequate nutrition.

Each special situation requires individualized attention and support. Consulting with healthcare professionals, lactation consultants, and seeking guidance from support groups or online communities can provide invaluable assistance in navigating these unique breastfeeding challenges. Remember, with the right support and information, many special situations can still lead to a positive breastfeeding experience for both parent and baby.

PREMATURE BABIES AND NICU CARE

Premature babies, those born before 37 weeks of gestation, often require care in the Neonatal Intensive Care Unit (NICU) due to their unique medical needs and developmental immaturity. Breastfeeding and providing expressed breast milk play a crucial role in supporting the health and development of premature babies. Here's an expanded explanation of managing breastfeeding and NICU care for premature babies:

Initiating Breast Milk Production:

- **Early Expression of Breast Milk:** Begin expressing breast milk as soon as possible after delivery, even if the baby is not yet able to breastfeed. Frequent pumping sessions (every 2-3 hours) help establish and maintain milk supply.
- **Hospital-Grade Breast Pump:** Utilize a hospital-grade electric breast pump, which is effective in stimulating milk production and can be provided by the NICU or lactation consultant.

Establishing Breastfeeding in the NICU:

- **Kangaroo Care**: Practice kangaroo care, where the baby is held skin-to-skin against the parent's chest. This promotes bonding, regulates the baby's temperature, and enhances breastfeeding cues.
- **Oral Care and Suck Training**: NICU staff will assess the baby's readiness for oral feeding and provide oral care, such as gently rubbing the baby's gums and tongue. They will also guide parents on practicing non-nutritive sucking to develop the baby's sucking reflex.

- **Nipple Shields or Preemie Nipples**: For babies with difficulty latching, a lactation consultant or NICU staff may recommend using nipple shields or specialized preemie nipples to facilitate feeding.
- **Breastfeeding Education and Support**: Seek guidance from the NICU's lactation consultant, who can provide education on breastfeeding techniques, positioning, and addressing challenges specific to premature babies.

Transitioning to Exclusive Breastfeeding:

- **Gradual Introduction**: Initially, the baby may receive expressed breast milk through a feeding tube or bottle. As the baby's coordination and strength improve, breastfeeding can be gradually introduced, starting with short nursing sessions and progressing to full feeds at the breast.
- **Combination Feeding**: In some cases, a combination of breastfeeding and bottle-feeding may be necessary, allowing for easier monitoring of the baby's intake and facilitating weight gain.
- **Pace Feeding**: Encourage slow and paced feeding when using a bottle, mimicking the natural rhythm of breastfeeding, to avoid overfeeding and support the baby's ability to transition between breast and bottle.

Pumping and Storing Breast Milk:

- Proper Pumping Technique: Ensure proper breast pumping technique, including using the correct flange size, maintaining a regular pumping schedule, and ensuring cleanliness of equipment.
- Storage and Handling: Follow guidelines for storing and handling breast milk provided by the NICU or lactation consultant. Label each container with the date and time of expression and use the oldest milk first.

Emotional Support and Self-Care:

- **Seek Emotional Support**: Coping with the NICU experience can be emotionally challenging. Seek emotional support from healthcare providers, counselors, support groups, or online communities specifically tailored for parents of premature babies.
- **Self-Care**: Take care of your physical and emotional well-being by getting adequate rest, eating nutritious meals, and engaging in activities that help you relax and recharge.

Remember, every premature baby's journey is unique, and the NICU staff, lactation consultants, and other healthcare professionals are there to provide guidance and support. With patience, persistence, and expert assistance, breastfeeding can be established and contribute to the baby's growth, development, and overall well-being.

BREASTFEEDING TWINS OR MULTIPLES

Breastfeeding twins or multiples can be a rewarding and fulfilling experience, although it may present some unique challenges. With proper support and strategies, it is absolutely possible to breastfeed multiple babies successfully. Here's an expanded explanation on managing breastfeeding for twins or multiples:

Establishing a Feeding Routine:

- **Frequent Feedings**: In the early days, aim to breastfeed your babies frequently, ideally every 2-3 hours, to meet their nutritional needs and stimulate milk production.
- **Simultaneous Feedings**: Try tandem breastfeeding, where you nurse both babies at the same time. This can help save time and ensure both babies receive equal attention.
- **Alternate Feedings**: Alternatively, you can choose to feed each baby separately, rotating between them for each feeding session. This allows for one-on-one bonding time with each

baby and can be helpful if one baby needs extra attention or has different feeding preferences.

Proper Positioning and Latching Techniques:

- Football Hold: The football hold, where each baby is positioned on a pillow at your sides with their bodies tucked under your arms, is commonly used for breastfeeding twins. This position provides good visibility and control over each baby's latch.
- Cradle Hold: The cradle hold, where each baby is cradled in one arm, can also be used. Use pillows for support, ensuring each baby is positioned securely and latched on correctly.
- Side-Lying Position: Breastfeeding while lying on your side can be comfortable and convenient, especially during nighttime feedings.

Support and Assistance:

- **Lactation Consultant**: Seek guidance from a lactation consultant experienced in working with multiples. They can provide personalized support, assess latch and positioning, and offer helpful tips and techniques.
- **Support Groups**: Join local support groups or online communities specifically for parents of

twins or multiples. Connecting with other parents going through similar experiences can provide valuable insights and encouragement.

Managing Milk Supply:

- **Breast Pumping**: Consider using a double electric breast pump to save time and ensure both breasts are adequately stimulated. Pumping between feedings can help boost milk supply and provide additional milk for future feedings.
- **Supplemental Feeding**: In some cases, supplementing with expressed breast milk or formula may be necessary to ensure all babies are receiving adequate nutrition, especially if your milk supply needs time to catch up with their needs.

Self-Care:

Rest and Nutrition: Take care of yourself by getting enough rest, eating nutritious meals, and staying hydrated. Remember that caring for multiple babies can be physically and emotionally demanding, so prioritize self-care.

Accept Help: Don't hesitate to accept help from family members, friends, or volunteers who can assist with household tasks or caring for the babies, allowing you to focus on breastfeeding and bonding.

Breastfeeding twins or multiples may require patience and flexibility, but with persistence, support, and proper techniques, it is possible to establish and maintain successful breastfeeding. Every baby is unique, so follow their cues and consult with healthcare professionals or lactation consultants as needed to address any specific challenges or concerns.

BREASTFEEDING AND MEDICATIONS

Breastfeeding and medications can go hand in hand, but it's important to be aware of the potential effects of medications on breast milk and the nursing baby. Here's an expanded explanation on breastfeeding and medications:

Consult with Healthcare Providers:

- **Healthcare Provider Guidance:** Before taking any medication while breastfeeding, consult with your healthcare provider, such as your doctor or pharmacist. They can provide specific information about the safety of medications for breastfeeding mothers.

- **Consideration of Individual Factors**: Factors such as the medication's safety profile, dosage, frequency of use, the age of the baby, and the overall health of both the mother and baby will be considered when determining the compatibility of a medication with breastfeeding.

Medication Categories:

- **Compatible Medications**: Many medications are considered safe to use while breastfeeding. These include certain antibiotics, pain relievers (such as acetaminophen), most asthma medications, and some antidepressants. However, it's crucial to consult with your healthcare provider to confirm the safety of a specific medication.
- **Medications to Use with Caution**: Some medications may require caution or additional monitoring while breastfeeding. These include certain antidepressants, antipsychotics, anticoagulants, and medications with sedating effects. Your healthcare provider can help assess the benefits versus potential risks and guide you accordingly.
- **Medications to Avoid**: There are some medications that are generally not recommended during breastfeeding due to their potential risks to the nursing baby. These may include

chemotherapy drugs, certain antiretroviral medications for HIV, and certain medications with a high risk of adverse effects.

Timing of Medication Administration:

Plan Medication Timing: Whenever possible, try to take medications immediately after breastfeeding or during a longer stretch between feedings to minimize the amount of medication present in breast milk during subsequent feedings.

Short Half-Life Medications: Some medications have a short half-life, meaning they are eliminated from the body relatively quickly. Taking these medications just before the baby's longest sleep period can reduce their exposure to the medication.

Monitoring the Baby:

- **Observe for Side Effects**: While taking medication, closely monitor your baby for any unusual changes, such as excessive drowsiness, irritability, poor feeding, or any other unexpected symptoms. If you notice any concerning signs, contact your healthcare provider promptly.
- **Monitor Milk Supply and Infant Growth**: Certain medications may have an impact on milk

supply. Keep track of your milk production and monitor your baby's growth and weight gain to ensure they are receiving adequate nutrition.

Alternative Medications or Dosages:

- **Explore Alternative Medications**: In some cases, your healthcare provider may recommend alternative medications that are considered safer during breastfeeding. Discuss potential alternatives and weigh the benefits and risks.
- **Dosage Adjustments**: For medications that are not entirely compatible with breastfeeding, your healthcare provider may suggest dosage adjustments or modifications to minimize the exposure of the medication to the baby.

Remember, the decision to take medication while breastfeeding should be made in collaboration with your healthcare provider. Open communication and accurate information about the specific medication and your breastfeeding goals are essential for making informed decisions that prioritize the health and well-being of both you and your baby.

Returning to work or school while breastfeeding can present challenges, but with proper planning and support, it is possible to continue breastfeeding successfully. Here's an expanded explanation on managing breastfeeding while returning to work or school:

Plan Ahead:

- **Pumping Schedule**: Establish a pumping schedule before returning to work or school. Start pumping a few weeks in advance to build up a supply of expressed breast milk and become familiar with the pumping routine.
- **Pumping Equipment**: Invest in a high-quality double electric breast pump and ensure you have all the necessary accessories, such as storage bags or bottles, cooler bags, and a clean and private space for pumping.
- **Communicate with Employers or School Administration**: Inform your employer or school administration about your intention to continue breastfeeding and discuss the accommodations they can provide, such as designated pumping breaks, a private pumping area, or flexible work or class schedules.

Storing and Transporting Breast Milk:

- **Proper Storage**: Follow guidelines for storing breast milk. Label each container with the date and time of expression, and use the oldest milk first. Store milk in a clean and dedicated space in the refrigerator or freezer.
- **Transporting Breast Milk**: Use insulated cooler bags with ice packs to transport expressed milk from home to work or school. Ensure the milk remains at a safe temperature during transportation.

Pumping at Work or School:

- **Establish a Routine**: Schedule regular pumping breaks throughout the day to maintain milk supply and prevent discomfort. Aim to pump every 3-4 hours, or as often as your baby would typically nurse.
- **Find a Suitable Pumping Space**: Seek out a private and clean space where you can comfortably pump. This can be an office, a lactation room, or a designated area provided by your employer or school. Advocate for a suitable space if one is not readily available.
- **Hands-Free Pumping**: Consider using a hands-free pumping bra or pumping bra attachment that

allows you to multitask while pumping, making it easier to work or study during your pumping sessions.

Nursing When Together:

Nurse on Demand: When you are with your baby, nurse on demand to maintain the breastfeeding relationship and strengthen the bond. This includes morning, evening, and nighttime feedings, as well as feeding during weekends and days off.

Seek Support:

- **Lactation Consultant:** Consult with a lactation consultant to address any concerns or challenges related to breastfeeding while returning to work or school. They can provide guidance on pumping techniques, maintaining milk supply, and troubleshooting any issues that arise.
- **Support Groups:** Connect with other breastfeeding parents who are navigating similar situations. Support groups or online communities can provide valuable advice, encouragement, and a sense of camaraderie.

Remember, transitioning back to work or school while breastfeeding requires patience, organization, and support. Be flexible and prepared to make adjustments along the way. With proper planning and a supportive environment, you can continue to provide the benefits of breastfeeding to your baby while pursuing your professional or educational goals.

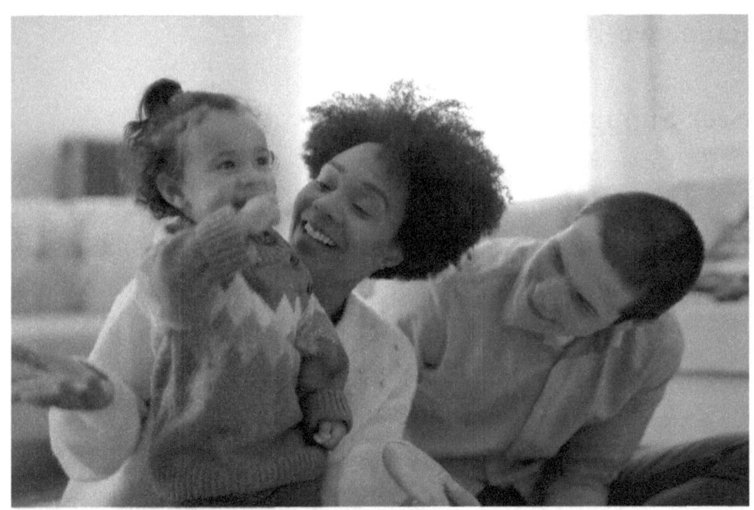

CHAPTER 6

WEANING AND EXTENDED BREASTFEEDING

Weaning and extended breastfeeding are important aspects of a breastfeeding journey. Here's an expanded explanation of weaning and extended breastfeeding:

Weaning:

- **Introduction of Complementary Foods**: Around six months of age, infants can begin exploring solid foods while continuing to breastfeed. This gradual introduction of complementary foods is a natural transition towards weaning.
- **Baby-Led Weaning**: Baby-led weaning involves allowing the baby to self-feed and explore a variety of foods at their own pace, while still maintaining breastfeeding as a source of nutrition and comfort.
- **Gradual Weaning**: Weaning can be a gradual process, where breastfeeding sessions are gradually reduced or replaced with alternative sources of nutrition, such as formula or solid foods.

- **Baby's Cues**: Pay attention to your baby's cues and readiness for weaning. Some babies naturally become less interested in breastfeeding as they grow and become more independent.

Emotional and Physical Considerations:

- **Emotional Transition:** Weaning can be an emotional process for both the baby and the breastfeeding parent. It may be helpful to offer additional comfort, cuddles, and attention during this transition period.
- **Gradual Adjustment:** Gradual weaning allows the body to gradually decrease milk production, reducing the risk of engorgement or mastitis. If weaning abruptly, it's important to manage milk supply changes to minimize discomfort or potential complications.
- **Hormonal Changes:** Weaning can result in hormonal shifts, potentially affecting mood and emotions. Being aware of these changes and seeking support from loved ones or healthcare professionals can be beneficial.

Extended Breastfeeding:

- **Benefits of Extended Breastfeeding:** Extended breastfeeding refers to continuing to breastfeed beyond the first year and into toddlerhood or even longer. Extended breastfeeding offers continued nutritional and immunological benefits, enhanced bonding, and comfort for both the child and the breastfeeding parent.

- **Child-Led Weaning:** Some families choose to let the child lead the weaning process, allowing them to self-wean when they are ready. This can be a gentle and gradual approach, respecting the child's needs and preferences.
- **Cultural and Personal Perspectives:** The decision to practice extended breastfeeding is personal and influenced by cultural, social, and individual factors. It's important to respect and support the choices made by each family regarding the duration of breastfeeding.

Transitioning to Alternative Forms of Nutrition:

- **Nutritional Needs:** As the child grows, their nutritional needs expand beyond breast milk. Introduce a variety of healthy foods to provide a well-balanced diet and meet their nutritional requirements.
- **Alternative Sources of Comfort:** As breastfeeding decreases, alternative sources of comfort, such as cuddling, gentle rocking, or offering a favorite blanket or toy, can help the

child adjust to the decrease in breastfeeding sessions.

- **Maintaining Bonding and Connection:** Although breastfeeding may decrease, maintaining a strong bond and connection with your child is crucial. Spend quality time together, engage in interactive play, and provide nurturing and affection through other means.

Seeking Support:

Lactation Consultant or Support Groups: If you have questions or concerns about weaning or extended breastfeeding, consult with a lactation consultant or seek support from breastfeeding support groups. They can provide guidance, encouragement, and evidence-based information to support your choices.

Remember, weaning and extended breastfeeding are personal decisions that should be based on the needs and desires of both the child and the breastfeeding parent. It's important to approach these transitions with patience, flexibility, and support, ensuring the well-being and comfort of both you and your child.

SIGNS OF READINESS FOR WEANING

Knowing when your child is ready for weaning is an important aspect of the breastfeeding journey. Here are some signs that indicate your child may be ready to start the weaning process:

Age and Developmental Milestones:

- **Introducing Solid Foods:** Around six months of age, most babies are developmentally ready to begin exploring solid foods. This can be an indication that they are ready to transition from exclusive breastfeeding to a combination of breastfeeding and solid foods.
- **Increased Independence:** As babies grow older, they become more independent and curious about their surroundings. They may start showing interest in exploring new tastes, textures, and self-feeding, which can be a sign of readiness for weaning.

Decreased Interest in Breastfeeding:

- **Shortened Nursing Sessions:** If your child begins to nurse for shorter durations during each feeding session or loses interest in breastfeeding altogether, it may be a sign that they are ready to wean.

- **Self-Directed Weaning:** Some children naturally start self-weaning by decreasing their interest in breastfeeding and showing a preference for other sources of nutrition and comfort.

Introduction of Other Food and Drinks:

- **Acceptance of Solid Foods:** When your child starts accepting and enjoying a variety of solid foods, it indicates that they are expanding their palate and becoming more open to alternative sources of nutrition.
- **Interest in Drinking from Cups:** If your child shows curiosity about drinking from a cup and successfully sips from it, it can indicate their readiness to transition from breastfeeding to cup feeding.

Increased Independence and Self-Soothing:

- **Self-Soothing Techniques:** If your child starts using other self-soothing techniques, such as using a pacifier, sucking their thumb, or finding comfort in a favorite blanket or toy, it suggests they are becoming more independent and finding alternative ways to soothe themselves.
- **Easily Distracted During Breastfeeding:** If your child becomes easily distracted during

breastfeeding sessions and frequently breaks the latch to explore their surroundings, it may be a sign that they are becoming less reliant on breastfeeding for comfort and nourishment.

Emotional and Behavioral Cues:

- **Contentment after Feeding:** If your child consistently appears satisfied and content after a breastfeeding session and does not exhibit signs of hunger shortly afterward, it can indicate that they are receiving adequate nutrition from other sources and are ready for gradual weaning.
- **Interest in Interacting with Others:** As children grow, their social interactions and interest in engaging with others increase. If your child becomes more eager to engage with family members, playmates, or siblings, it may indicate that they are ready to transition away from breastfeeding as their primary source of connection and comfort.

It's important to note that every child is different, and readiness for weaning can vary. Pay attention to your child's cues, developmental milestones, and individual needs when considering the appropriate time to start the weaning process. Consult with a healthcare professional or a lactation consultant for personalized guidance and support during this transition.

INTRODUCING SOLID FOODS

Introducing solid foods is an exciting milestone in your baby's development. Here's an expanded explanation on how to introduce solid foods to your baby:

Timing:

- **Age Recommendations:** The American Academy of Pediatrics (AAP) recommends introducing solid foods around six months of age. By this time, babies have typically developed the necessary skills, such as head control and the ability to sit with support, to begin exploring solid foods.
- **Signs of Readiness:** Look for signs of readiness, such as good head control, ability to sit with support, showing interest in food, and being able to move food from the front of the mouth to the back (tongue thrust reflex starts to diminish).

Types of Foods:

- **Start with Single-Ingredient Foods:** Begin with single-ingredient, pureed or mashed foods to identify any possible allergies or sensitivities. Good options include pureed fruits (such as apples, pears, or bananas), vegetables (such as sweet potatoes, carrots, or peas), and iron-fortified baby cereals (such as rice, oatmeal, or barley).

- **Introduce New Foods Slowly:** Introduce new foods one at a time, with a few days in between each new food. This allows you to monitor for any adverse reactions or allergies.
- **Gradual Texture Changes:** As your baby becomes more comfortable with purees, gradually introduce thicker textures and soft, mashed foods to encourage chewing and development of oral motor skills.

Feeding Techniques:

- **Feeding Schedule:** Start with one or two small meals per day, gradually increasing to three meals as your baby shows interest and appetite. Breast milk or formula should still be the primary source of nutrition during the first year.
- **Responsive Feeding:** Allow your baby to guide the pace and amount of food consumed. Watch for hunger and fullness cues, and never force-feed your baby.

- **Offer a Variety of Foods:** Introduce a wide range of fruits, vegetables, whole grains, and proteins to expose your baby to different flavors and textures. This helps establish healthy eating habits and exposes them to a variety of nutrients.
- **Encourage Self-Feeding:** As your baby develops their motor skills, introduce finger foods that are soft and age-appropriate, such as small pieces of cooked vegetables, soft fruits, or well-cooked pasta. This encourages self-feeding and improves hand-eye coordination.

Food Preparation and Safety:

- **Food Consistency:** In the beginning, puree or mash foods to a smooth and thin consistency. As your baby becomes more skilled at eating, you can gradually increase the texture to match their abilities.
- **Safe Food Choices:** Avoid offering foods that are choking hazards, such as whole grapes, nuts, popcorn, or chunks of meat. Cut food into small, bite-sized pieces or offer it in a mashed or pureed form.
- **Hygiene and Storage:** Practice good hygiene when preparing and serving food. Wash hands thoroughly, clean utensils and surfaces, and store

prepared baby food in airtight containers in the refrigerator for a limited time.

- **Allergenic Foods:** Introduce allergenic foods, such as peanuts, tree nuts, eggs, fish, and shellfish, one at a time and in small quantities. Discuss any concerns about food allergies with your pediatrician.

Breastfeeding or Formula Feeding:

- **Continue Breastfeeding or Formula Feeding:** Solid foods should complement, not replace, breast milk or formula as the main source of nutrition for the first year. Offer breast milk or formula before offering solid foods to ensure that your baby receives adequate nutrition.
- **Feeding Sequence:** Initially, breastfeed or offer a bottle before offering solid foods to satisfy your baby's hunger. As solid food intake increases, you can adjust the sequence based on your baby's needs and preferences

GRADUAL WEANING STRATEGIES

Gradual weaning allows both you and your baby to transition from breastfeeding to alternative sources of nutrition and comfort in a gentle and supportive manner. Here are some strategies for gradual weaning:

Slowly Replace Breastfeedings:

- **Choose One Feeding at a Time:** Start by replacing one breastfeeding session with a bottle of expressed breast milk or formula. Select a feeding that is least important to you or your baby, such as a midday feeding.
- **Maintain Other Breastfeedings:** Continue breastfeeding for the remaining feedings in the day to provide familiarity and comfort to your baby while gradually reducing the number of breastfeedings

.

Offer Alternatives:

- **Introduce Bottles:** If your baby hasn't already been introduced to bottles, gradually introduce them as you replace breastfeedings. Start with small amounts of expressed breast milk or formula in a bottle and gradually increase the amount over time.
- **Cup or Sippy Cup:** As your baby becomes proficient at drinking from a cup, you can gradually transition from bottles to cup or sippy cup feedings for the replaced breastfeedings.
- **Solid Foods:** As your baby's intake of solid foods increases, offer them as an alternative source of nutrition alongside breast milk or formula.

Shorten the Duration of Breastfeedings:

- **Encourage Efficient Feeding:** Encourage your baby to nurse more efficiently by making sure they have a proper latch and ensuring they are actively nursing. This can help reduce the duration of breastfeeding sessions and gradually wean them from extended comfort nursing.
- **Distractions and Diversions:** Engage your baby in activities, play, or offer toys during breastfeeding sessions to help distract them and gradually reduce the length of each feeding.

Gradual Time Spacing:

Increase Time Between Feedings: Gradually increase the time between breastfeedings. For example, if you typically breastfeed every two hours, extend it to two and a half hours, then three hours, and so on. This allows your baby to adapt to longer intervals without breastfeeding.

Comfort and Reassurance:

- **Cuddle and Bonding:** As you reduce breastfeeding sessions, make sure to provide extra cuddling, skin-to-skin contact, and bonding time with your baby. This helps them feel secure and loved during the transition.

- **Offer Alternative Comfort:** Introduce other comforting techniques, such as rocking, singing, gentle massages, or providing a special blanket or toy, to help ease the transition from breastfeeding.

Support and Patience:

- Emotional Support: Weaning can be an emotional process for both you and your baby. Seek support from your partner, family, or friends to help you through the transition.
- Be Patient and Flexible: Every child is different, and weaning may take longer for some than others. Be patient and flexible, adjusting the pace of weaning to suit your baby's needs and comfort.

Remember, gradual weaning is a personal process, and the timeline and strategies may vary for each family. Listen to your baby's cues, follow their lead, and make adjustments accordingly. If you have concerns or questions, consult with a healthcare professional or lactation consultant for guidance and support throughout the weaning journey.

CHAPTER 7

EXTENDED BREASTFEEDING BENEFITS AND CONSIDERATIONS

Extended breastfeeding, which refers to breastfeeding beyond the first year and into toddlerhood or even longer, can offer numerous benefits for both the child and the breastfeeding parent. Here are some expanded benefits and considerations of extended breastfeeding:

Benefits for the Child:

- **Continued Nutrition and Immune Support**: Breast milk remains a valuable source of nutrition for toddlers, providing essential nutrients, vitamins, and antibodies that support their growth, development, and immune system.
- **Enhanced Brain Development**: Breast milk contains important fatty acids, such as DHA (docosahexaenoic acid), which contribute to optimal brain development and cognitive function in toddlers.
- **Reduced Risk of Illness**: Breast milk continues to offer protection against various infections, allergies, respiratory illnesses, and

gastrointestinal disorders, helping to reduce the risk and severity of these conditions.

- **Emotional Comfort and Bonding**: Breastfeeding nurtures the emotional bond between the child and the breastfeeding parent, providing comfort, security, and a sense of closeness and connection.

Benefits for the Breastfeeding Parent:

- **Emotional Bonding and Relaxation**: Extended breastfeeding fosters a strong emotional bond between the breastfeeding parent and the child, promoting a sense of closeness, security, and emotional well-being for both.
- **Hormonal Benefits:** Breastfeeding stimulates the release of oxytocin, a hormone that promotes feelings of relaxation, stress reduction, and bonding. Extended breastfeeding allows the continued experience of these hormonal benefits.
- **Reduced Risk of Certain Health Conditions**: Studies suggest that extended breastfeeding may contribute to a decreased risk of certain health conditions for the breastfeeding parent, such as breast and ovarian cancers, osteoporosis, and cardiovascular diseases.
- **Convenience and Cost-Effectiveness**: Extended breastfeeding eliminates the need for formula

preparation and reduces the cost of purchasing infant formula, bottles, and other feeding supplies.

Considerations for Extended Breastfeeding:

- **Nutritional Supplements**: As the child grows and their nutritional needs expand, it may be necessary to introduce complementary solid foods to ensure they receive a balanced diet that meets their nutritional requirements.
- **Nutrient-Dense Foods**: As breastfeeding continues, it's important for the breastfeeding parent to prioritize their own nutrition by consuming a well-balanced diet with nutrient-dense foods to support their own health and energy levels.
- **Supportive Social Environment**: Extended breastfeeding may face some societal challenges and misconceptions. It's important to create a supportive social environment that respects and understands the benefits and choices of extended breastfeeding.
- **Individual Needs and Preferences:** Every family and child is unique, and the decision to practice extended breastfeeding should be based on the individual needs, preferences, and

circumstances of both the child and the breastfeeding parent.

It's important to remember that the decision to engage in extended breastfeeding is a personal one, influenced by cultural, social, and individual factors. It should be made with careful consideration of the well-being and comfort of both the child and the breastfeeding parent. Seeking support from healthcare professionals, lactation consultants, and breastfeeding support groups can provide guidance, information, and encouragement throughout the extended breastfeeding journey.

BREASTFEEDING AND SPECIAL CIRCUMSTANCES

Breastfeeding is a natural and beneficial way to nourish and bond with your baby. However, certain special circumstances may arise that can impact breastfeeding. Here are some expanded considerations and strategies for breastfeeding in special circumstances:

Multiple Births (Twins, Triplets, etc.):

- **Establishing Milk Supply**: Multiple babies have higher nutritional demands, so establishing a plentiful milk supply is crucial. Frequent breastfeeding or pumping sessions, including cluster feeding, can help stimulate milk production.

- **Positioning and Support**: Experiment with different breastfeeding positions to accommodate multiple babies simultaneously. Seek assistance from a lactation consultant or support group experienced in breastfeeding multiples.
- **Supplementation if Needed**: In some cases, supplementation with expressed breast milk or formula may be necessary to ensure all babies receive adequate nutrition.

Premature or Ill Babies:

- **Kangaroo Care**: Skin-to-skin contact is highly beneficial for premature or ill babies. It helps regulate body temperature, promotes bonding, and enhances breastfeeding success.
- **Pumping and Milk Expression**: Initially, babies may be unable to breastfeed directly. Pumping breast milk and providing it through a bottle or tube feeding can ensure they receive the benefits of breast milk.
- **Support from Healthcare Providers**: Collaborate with the neonatal care team to develop a breastfeeding plan tailored to your baby's specific needs. Seek guidance from lactation consultants with experience in

supporting breastfeeding for premature or ill infants.

Adoption or Surrogacy:

- **Induced Lactation:** Through a process of hormonal stimulation and frequent breast stimulation, some non-birthing parents can induce lactation to breastfeed their adopted or surrogate-born baby. Working with a healthcare provider and lactation consultant is essential in this process.
- **Supplemental Feeding Methods:** In cases where induced lactation is not feasible, supplementing with donor milk or formula while engaging in skin-to-skin contact and breastfeeding attempts can still foster bonding and provide nutritional benefits.

Maternal Health Conditions:

- **Medications and Breastfeeding:** Consult with your healthcare provider to determine the compatibility of any medications you are taking with breastfeeding. In many cases, there are safe alternatives that allow you to continue breastfeeding.

- **Special Dietary Considerations:** Some maternal health conditions may require dietary modifications. Work with a registered dietitian or healthcare provider to ensure you are meeting your nutritional needs while breastfeeding.

Relactation:

Relactation refers to the process of restarting breastfeeding after a period of interruption. It can be useful if breastfeeding was discontinued temporarily due to factors such as medical procedures or inadequate milk supply.

Support and Patience: Seek guidance from a lactation consultant or breastfeeding support group to develop a relactation plan. It often involves frequent breastfeeding or pumping sessions, proper latch techniques, and addressing any underlying issues that led to the interruption.

Remember, each special circumstance is unique, and it's essential to seek personalized support from healthcare professionals, lactation consultants, and support groups. They can provide tailored guidance, address specific concerns, and offer strategies to overcome challenges in order to optimize breastfeeding success in special circumstances.

ADOPTION AND INDUCED LACTATION

Adoption and induced lactation provide an opportunity for non-birthing parents to breastfeed their adopted child. While it may require additional effort and preparation, it can be a rewarding experience that promotes bonding and provides nutritional benefits. Here's an expanded explanation of adoption and induced lactation:

Adoption and Breastfeeding:

- **Benefits of Breastfeeding:** Breastfeeding offers numerous benefits, including immune system support, optimal nutrition, and emotional bonding between parent and child. It can enhance the attachment process and provide comfort and security to the adopted child.
- **Supplemental Feeding:** In cases where the non-birthing parent is unable to produce sufficient breast milk, supplemental feeding with donor milk or formula can be incorporated while still engaging in breastfeeding for emotional and bonding purposes.

Induced Lactation:

Induced lactation is the process of stimulating lactation in a non-pregnant individual. It involves mimicking the hormonal changes that occur during pregnancy and breastfeeding to encourage milk production.

- **Preparation and Timing:** The process of induced lactation typically begins several months before the expected breastfeeding start date. This allows time for hormonal stimulation and milk production to occur.

- **Working with Healthcare Providers:** Consulting with healthcare providers, such as lactation consultants and medical professionals familiar with induced lactation, is crucial for guidance and support throughout the process.

- **Hormonal Stimulation:** Hormonal therapy, such as using medications like birth control pills or hormone replacement therapy, may be prescribed to simulate pregnancy and initiate milk production.

- **Breast Stimulation:** Regular breast stimulation through manual expression, breast pumping, or the use of a supplemental nursing system (SNS) helps signal the body to produce milk. This can be done several times a day to increase milk production gradually.

- **Galactagogues:** Some individuals may use galactagogues, which are substances believed to promote milk production. Common examples include fenugreek, blessed thistle, and lactation teas. However, their efficacy varies, and it's important to consult with healthcare professionals before using them.

- **Support and Patience:** Induced lactation can be a challenging and time-consuming process. It requires patience, dedication, and support from healthcare providers, partners, and support groups who can offer guidance, encouragement, and emotional support.

Supplementation and Breastfeeding Support:

- **Supplemental Feeding:** In cases where induced lactation does not result in a full milk supply, supplementing breastfeeding sessions with donor milk or formula ensures the baby receives adequate nutrition.
- **Latch and Positioning Techniques:** Learning proper latch and positioning techniques from a lactation consultant can help maximize milk transfer and promote successful breastfeeding sessions.
- **Breastfeeding Support:** Seeking support from lactation consultants, breastfeeding support groups, and online communities can provide valuable information, guidance, and emotional support throughout the breastfeeding journey.

It's important to note that every individual's response to induced lactation may vary. While some non-birthing parents may be able to achieve a full milk supply, others may experience partial milk production. Regardless of the outcome, the act of breastfeeding itself can strengthen the bond between parent and child. Ultimately, the well-being and happiness of both the parent and child should guide the decisions made regarding adoption and induced lactation.

RELACTATION AFTER A GAP

Relactation is the process of reestablishing breastfeeding after a period of interruption, such as when breastfeeding was discontinued temporarily due to various reasons. It involves stimulating milk production again and rebuilding the breastfeeding relationship between parent and child. Here's an expanded explanation of relactation after a gap:

Motivation and Support:

- **Personal Motivation:** A strong desire and commitment to relactate are essential for success. Identifying your reasons for wanting to breastfeed again can provide the motivation needed to overcome challenges.

- **Partner and Family Support:** Having the support of your partner and family members can significantly contribute to your emotional well-being and provide practical assistance throughout the relactation process.

Establishing Milk Supply:

- **Frequent Breast Stimulation:** Increasing breast stimulation through breastfeeding, pumping, or a combination of both is crucial for stimulating milk production. Aim for frequent sessions, ideally every 2-3 hours, including nighttime feedings.
- **Effective Breast Pumping:** If direct breastfeeding is not possible or if the baby is not yet latching, using a high-quality breast pump can help maintain regular breast stimulation and stimulate milk production.
- **Skin-to-Skin Contact:** Skin-to-skin contact with your baby, often referred to as kangaroo care, can help stimulate milk production and promote the bonding process.
- **Breast Massage and Compression:** Gentle breast massage and compression during breastfeeding or pumping sessions can aid in milk flow and emptying the breasts more effectively.

- **Galactagogues:** Some lactation consultants or healthcare providers may recommend the use of galactagogues, such as fenugreek or blessed thistle, to help support milk production. However, it's important to consult with a healthcare professional before using any herbal remedies.

Latching and Breastfeeding Techniques:

- **Latching Assistance:** Seek guidance from a lactation consultant to ensure a proper latch. They can help assess the baby's latch, positioning, and suckling pattern to optimize milk transfer.
- **Breastfeeding Positions:** Experiment with different breastfeeding positions to find the most comfortable and effective one for you and your baby. Various positions, such as the cradle hold or football hold, can facilitate a successful latch.
- **Skin-to-Skin Contact:** Skin-to-skin contact during breastfeeding helps establish a nurturing and secure environment, promotes bonding, and encourages the baby's instinctual feeding behaviors.

Supplemental Feeding:

While relactation is in progress, it may be necessary to supplement breastfeeding sessions with expressed breast milk or formula to ensure the baby receives adequate nutrition. This can be done using a cup, spoon, syringe, or a supplemental nursing system (SNS) that delivers additional milk while breastfeeding

.

Persistence and Patience:

Relactation is a process that takes time and patience. It's important to be patient with yourself and your baby as you both adjust to the reestablishment of breastfeeding. Results may vary, but even small amounts of breast milk can provide nutritional and emotional benefits.

Seek Support: Reach out to lactation consultants, breastfeeding support groups, and online communities to seek guidance, share experiences, and receive emotional support throughout the relactation journey.

Remember, every breastfeeding journey is unique, and relactation success can vary. Celebrate each milestone and progress made along the way, whether it's a few drops of milk or the baby successfully latching. The bond and nurturing provided through the relactation process can be meaningful and beneficial for both parent and child.

Donor Milk and Milk Banking

Donor milk and milk banking provide a valuable resource for babies who are unable to receive breast milk directly from their own mothers. Whether due to medical conditions, prematurity, or other circumstances, donor milk can offer numerous benefits. Here's an expanded explanation of donor milk and milk banking:

Donor Milk:

Donor milk refers to breast milk that is generously provided by lactating individuals who have excess milk and willingly choose to donate it to support other babies' health and well-being.

- **Nutritional Composition:** Donor milk is similar in composition to a mother's own milk, providing essential nutrients, antibodies, enzymes, and growth factors that support a baby's growth and development.
- **Pasteurization:** To ensure safety and minimize the risk of transmitting infections, donated milk goes through a process of pasteurization. This involves heating the milk to eliminate potential pathogens while preserving its nutritional and immunological properties.

- **Accessibility:** Donor milk is typically made available through human milk banks or milk sharing networks, which follow strict guidelines for collection, screening, processing, and distribution.

Human Milk Banks:

- **Milk Bank Operations:** Human milk banks are facilities that collect, process, store, and distribute donor milk to infants in need. They adhere to rigorous protocols to ensure the safety and quality of the donated milk.
- **Donor Screening:** Donor milk banks have comprehensive screening processes in place to assess the health and lifestyle of potential donors. This includes health history questionnaires, blood tests, and interviews to ensure the milk is safe for consumption.
- **Pasteurization and Storage:** Donated milk undergoes pasteurization to eliminate potential pathogens while preserving its nutritional value. After pasteurization, the milk is stored in sterile containers and frozen until it is needed.
- **Prescription and Distribution:** Healthcare professionals, such as doctors or lactation consultants, typically prescribe donor milk for infants who require it. Milk banks work closely

with healthcare providers to ensure appropriate distribution based on the specific needs of each recipient.

Benefits and Considerations:

- **Premature and Medically Fragile Infants:** Donor milk is especially beneficial for premature infants who may face challenges in digesting formula or have a higher risk of infection. The protective factors in breast milk can help reduce the incidence of serious complications in these vulnerable infants.
- **Improved Health Outcomes:** Research suggests that receiving donor milk is associated with reduced rates of necrotizing enterocolitis (NEC), a severe intestinal condition, and other gastrointestinal and respiratory infections.
- **Emotional and Psychological Benefits:** For families who are unable to provide breast milk, having access to donor milk can alleviate feelings of guilt or inadequacy and allow them to provide their baby with the benefits of breast milk.
- **Safety and Quality Assurance:** Human milk banks adhere to strict guidelines for donor screening, milk processing, and storage to ensure the safety and quality of the donated milk. This includes pasteurization, bacterial testing, and thorough record-keeping.

Milk Sharing Networks:

Informal milk sharing networks involve direct sharing of breast milk between individuals without the involvement of a formal milk bank. It's important to note that milk obtained through informal networks carries additional risks, such as inadequate screening and potential contamination.

If you're considering using donor milk for your baby, consult with healthcare professionals, such as pediatricians or lactation consultants, who can guide you through the process and help you find reputable milk banks or networks. They can provide information about the benefits, risks, and proper usage of donor milk based on your specific circumstances.

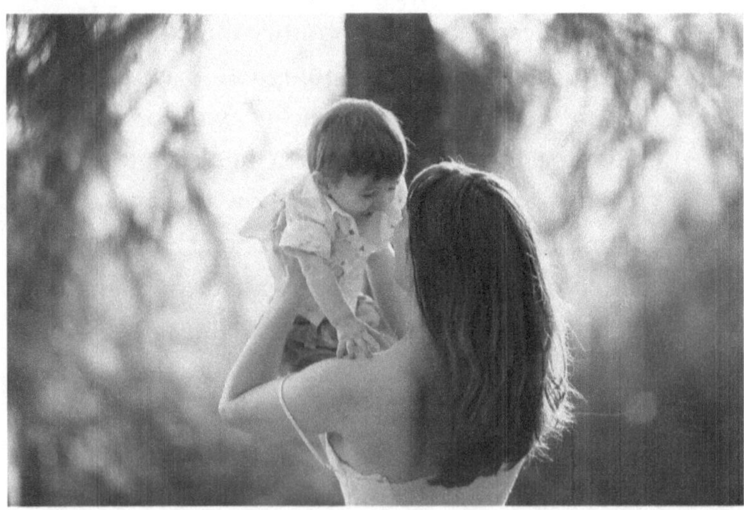